Physiological Society Study Guides   Number 1

Acid-base balance

Physiological Society Study Guides

1 **Acid-base balance**
    edited by R. Hainsworth

Forthcoming

Amino acid transport
Respiration

Physiological Society Study Guides   *Number 1*

Acid-base balance

Edited by
R. Hainsworth

Manchester University Press

Published by Manchester University Press
Oxford Road, Manchester M13 9PL, UK
and 27 South Main Street, Wolfeboro, N.H. 03894-2069, USA

British Library cataloguing in publication data
Acid–base balance. — (Physiological Society
   study guides; no. 1)
   1. Acid–base equilibrium
   I. Hainsworth, R.   II. Series
   612'.01522   QP90.7

Library of Congress cataloging in publication data applied for

ISBN 0 7190 1981 8 hardback
ISBN 0 7190 1982 6 paperback

Typeset in Hong Kong
by Graphicraft Typesetters Ltd., Hong Kong

Printed and bound in Great Britain by
Biddles Ltd, Guildford and King's Lynn

Contents

Foreword   vii

List of contributors   ix

1 **The physical chemistry of acid–base balance**
   1.1 why is acid–base balance important?   1
   1.2 Buffers (short-term control of pH)   3
   1.3 Buffer systems in the body   13
   1.4 Buffering power of blood components   20
   1.5 Further aspects of the bicarbonate buffer system   21
   1.6 Renal regulation of acid–base balance   26
   1.7 Further reading   26

2 **Renal control of acid–base balance**
   2.1 Introduction   27
   2.2 The source of excreted hydrogen ions   29
   2.3 Reabsorption of filtered bicarbonate   31
   2.4 Urinary acidification and the restoration of depleted
       bicarbonate   39
   2.5 Renal compensation of respiratory acid–base
       disturbances   44
   2.6 Potassium and acid–base balance   46
   2.7 Bicarbonate, chloride and the 'anion gap'   47
   2.8 Sodium, diuretics and acid–base balance   47
   2.9 Further reading   48

3 **Intracellular pH**
   3.1 Introduction   50
   3.2 Methods for measuring pH_i 50
   3.3 Are H^+ ions passively distributed?   53
   3.4 External influences on pH_i 55

3.5 Intracellular buffering 59
3.6 Intracellular pH regulation 62
3.7 Intracellular pH changes in ischaemia, acidosis and
    alkalosis 66
3.8 The H^+ ion as an intracellular messenger 63
3.9 Further reading 72

4 **Acid–base control in the whole body**
4.1 Importance of acid–base control 75
4.2 Some definitions used in acid–base balance 76
4.3 Physiological consequences of acid–base
    disturbances 76
4.4 Buffering in the blood and extracellular fluid 78
4.5 Intracellular buffering 81
4.6 Whole body titration 82
4.7 Management of acute acid–base disorders 87
4.8 Estimation of blood pH and PCO_2 90
4.9 Further reading 94

5 **Acid–base balance for the clinician**
5.1 Introduction 96
5.2 History 96
5.3 Acids and bases 97
5.4 Buffers 98
5.5 The acid–base diagram 100
5.6 Respiratory acid–base disturbances 102
5.7 Metabolic acid–base disturbances 105
5.8 Clinical examples of the use of the acid–base
    diagram 107
5.9 Further reading 118

Appendix 1 Teaching material on acid–base balance 121

Appendix 2 Class experiments:
    pH regulation 123
    Urinary excretion of acids and alkalis: buffers 132

Appendix 3 Problems 146

Index 151

Foreword

'Acid–base balance' is the first of a series of study guides based on symposia organised by the Education Subcommittee of the Physiological Society. These symposia deal with topics which are found by students to be particularly difficult or confusing. Acid–base balance falls squarely into this category. This may partly be due to the tendency for it to be taught from so many different viewpoints: the account given in the renal physiology course tends to be different from that in the respiration course and the clinician tends to have yet another view. The difficulty and confusion are perhaps emphasised by the vast number of acid–base diagrams and nomograms which have been published.

This book, although based on a Physiological Society symposium, is not constrained by it. Indeed, two of the chapters were not covered at all by the symposium. It is aimed at undergraduate and postgraduate students as well as laboratory physiologists and those concerned with the management of patients with acid–base disorders.

The first chapter gives a description of the essential physical chemistry necessary for the understanding of the topic. This is presented in a way which will enable the reader to understand the mechanisms which apply. For example, the relative importances of the various buffer systems in the body are described and the reason why buffers operate best at pH values near to their pK is explained. The kidney is central to the long-term regulation of acid–base balance and the second chapter is devoted to a description of the excretion of acids and bases under various normal and abnormal conditions.

Recently there has been much interest in intracellular pH and its regulation. This is likely to be of increased importance as the new technique of nuclear magnetic resonance, which can estimate intracellular pH non-invasively, becomes more widely available. We have therefore devoted a chapter to the control of intracellular pH. Changes in pH_i are likely to be of importance in disease states and may be related to the growth of tumour cells. Intracellular pH may also be of great significance in normal physiology. For example, following fertilisation, there is an abrupt change in the pH of the egg and this may be related to its activation.

The last two chapters are concerned with acid–base control in the whole body and deal with whole body titration, short-term and long-term buffering and the clinical management of acid–base disorders. The clinical aspects are related to a simple acid–base diagram and are well illustrated by the use of very illuminating case histories.

In this book we attempt to merge several different approaches to acid–base balance although we have not tried to present a single simplified view of the topic and each chapter is intended to stand alone. Because the book is relatively short, the reader can readily compare the various approaches and this must enhance his or her understanding of the subject.

This book should be of wide interest and will fill a much needed gap. In addition to the text which should provide a readable and affordable account for students and their teachers, the appendices contain a list of available teaching material compiled by the Education Subcommittee which will be of use to those planning teaching courses, and a number of class experiments and problems.

R. Hainsworth

List of contributors

D. Attwell
Department of Physiology
University College
Gower Street
London

R. O. Law
Department of Physiology
The University
Leicester

R. C. Thomas
Department of Physiology
University of Bristol
University Walk
Bristol

R. Hainsworth
Department of Cardiovascular Studies
The University
Leeds

D. C. Flenley
Department of Respiratory Medicine
City Hospital
Greenbank Drive
Edinburgh

1

The physical chemistry of acid–base balance

D. Attwell   Department of Physiology, University College London

1.1 Why is acid–base balance important?

Evolutionary selection has produced several systems in the body which serve to keep the acidity of the body fluids within a rather narrow range. This allows more accurate control over cellular biochemistry than would otherwise be the case, because the rates of enzyme-catalysed reactions are usually strongly affected by changes in acidity. For example, changing the intracellular proton (H^+) concentration from $79 \times 10^{-9}\,mol \cdot l^{-1}$ to $63 \times 10^{-9}\,mol \cdot l^{-1}$, a pH change from 7.1 to 7.2 (see section 1.1.3 for a definition of pH), increases nearly twenty-fold the activity of phosphofructo-kinase, the key enzyme regulating the rate of glycolysis. Changes in acidity also have important effects on the excitability of the nervous system. In extreme cases, if the body becomes too acid the activity of the central nervous system is so depressed that death can occur from coma. Conversely, if the body becomes too alkaline, spontaneous action potentials produced in peripheral nerves can result in death from tetany (spasm) of the respiratory muscles.

This chapter provides the background in physical chemistry needed to understand how the body controls its acidity.

1.1.1 Sources of acid and alkali in the body

Many chemical reactions in the body produce or absorb protons. Dietary proteins and fats are converted to amino acids and fatty acids which circulate in the blood. Glucose, from dietary carbo-hydrate, is converted into pyruvic acid by the glycolytic pathway. Much larger amounts of H^+ can be formed indirectly from the

CO_2 generated by metabolism, which reacts with water to give H^+ and HCO_3^- (as will be described in detail in section 1.3.2). Extra acid loads are added to the blood by strenuous exercise (lactic acid is generated in the muscles to regenerate NAD^+, allowing glycolysis to continue when the oxygen supply is limited), and during diabetic ketosis (aceto-acetic acid and β-hydroxybutyric acid are generated as a result of massive fat breakdown). Dietary alkali is found in fruits, as the sodium and potassium salts of weak acids. On balance, people eating a typical western meat-containing diet generate an excess of H^+ in their bodies.

The excess CO_2 and H^+ generated in the body are ultimately removed by the lungs and kidneys, to keep the body H^+ level approximately constant. In the short term, various **buffer mechanisms** prevent the $[H^+]$ (H^+ concentration) changing too much. The buffers do not permanently get rid of excess H^+, they merely store it in a form which involves minimal changes in the free $[H^+]$. In this chapter, the short-term buffering carried out by weak acids is assessed from a theoretical viewpoint, to determine how buffering power depends on the concentration and buffering ability of the weak acid. This theory is then applied to assess the relative importance of different buffer systems in the blood. Finally, long-term control of acid–base balance by the lungs and kidney are discussed.

1.1.2 *Some useful definitions*

Neutral solution has its $[H^+]$ (actually $[H_3O^+]$) equal to its $[OH^-]$. For pure water at 25°C,

$$[H^+] \times [OH^-] = 10^{-14} (\text{mol} \cdot \text{l}^{-1})^2 \qquad (1.1)$$

and so for neutrality,

$$[H^+] = [OH^-] = 10^{-7} \text{mol} \cdot \text{l}^{-1} \text{ (M)}. \qquad (1.2)$$

The $[H^+]$ for neutrality is temperature-dependent. At 37°C the value is approximately $10^{-6.8} \text{mol} \cdot \text{l}^{-1}$.

Acid solutions have $[H^+]$ above the value for neutrality, e.g. $10^{-6} \text{mol} \cdot \text{l}^{-1}$.

Alkaline solutions have $[H^+]$ less than the value for neutrality, e.g. $10^{-8}\,mol\cdot l^{-1}$.

Acids are H^+ (H_3O^+) donors, e.g. $HCl \rightarrow H^+ + Cl^-$.

Bases are H^+ acceptors, e.g. $OH^- + H^+ \rightarrow H_2O$.

Strong acids are acids that dissociate essentially completely when added to neutral solution. For example, when HCl is added to water it dissociates almost completely into H^+ (i.e. H_3O^+) and Cl^- ions.

Weak acids are acids that dissociate only partially when the $[H^+]$ is near $10^{-7}\,mol\cdot l^{-1}$. For example when acetic acid (CH_3COOH) is added to water, although it partly dissociates into H^+ and CH_3COO^- ions, a significant fraction remains undissociated as CH_3COOH.

1.1.3 *Units for hydrogen ion concentration*

Since the concentration of hydrogen ions in most solutions is so small, it is convenient to define a new measure of acidity, the pH, as

$$pH = -\log_{10}[H^+] \qquad (1.3)$$

with $[H^+]$ in $mol\cdot l^{-1}$. Table 1.1 gives some examples of conversion from $[H^+]$ to pH notation, and a plot of eqn (1.3) is shown in Figure 1.1. A typical value for extracellular pH in humans is 7.4 (range 7.36–7.44) while intracellular pH is typically 7.0–7.2.

1.2 Buffers (short-term control of pH)

In this section the properties of buffer systems in general are described. The following section (1.3) applies this theory to buffers in the body.

1.2.1 *The Henderson–Hasselbalch equation*

Solutions containing weak acids can be used to reduce or 'buffer' changes in $[H^+]$ produced by adding acid or alkali. In the body buffering takes place in the blood, in the extracellular fluid and in the intracellular fluid. To understand how buffers work, consider a

Table 1.1. *Conversion of $[H^+]$ to pH.*

$[H^+]$	$1\,nmol \cdot l^{-1}$ $(10^{-9}\,mol \cdot l^{-1})$	$10\,nmol \cdot l^{-1}$	$40\,nmol \cdot l^{-1}$	$100\,nmol \cdot l^{-1}$	$1\,\mu mol \cdot l^{-1}$ $(10^{-6}\,mol \cdot l^{-1})$
pH	9	8	7.4	7	6

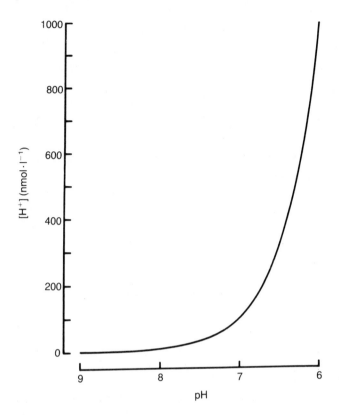

Fig. 1.1 The pH scale. A plot of equation (1.3) over the range of physiological interest. The $[H^+]$ scale on the ordinate is in $nmol \cdot l^{-1}$, where $1\,nmol \cdot l^{-1}$ is $10^{-9}\,mol \cdot l^{-1}$.

solution containing a weak acid, HA, and its salt, A^- ('A' might represent acetate, for example). The equilibrium between HA and A^- can be written

$$H^+ + A^- \underset{k_2}{\overset{k_1}{\rightleftharpoons}} HA \qquad (1.4)$$

where k_1 and k_2 are rate constants.
From the law of mass action, at equilibrium,

$$k_1[H^+][A^-] = k_2[HA] \tag{1.5}$$

or

$$[H^+] = K\frac{[HA]}{[A^-]} \tag{1.6}$$

where $K = k_2/k_1$ is the acid's dissociation constant. Taking logarithms (to base 10) we get

$$\log_{10}[H^+] = \log_{10} K + \log_{10}\frac{[HA]}{[A^-]} \tag{1.7}$$

or

$$-\log_{10}[H^+] = -\log_{10} K - \log_{10}\frac{[HA]}{[A^-]} \tag{1.8}$$

or

$$pH = pK + \log_{10}\frac{[A^-]}{[HA]} \tag{1.9}$$

where $pK = -\log_{10} K$.

Equation (1.9) is the Henderson–Hasselbalch equation, which we will use to investigate the relative importance of different buffers in the blood.

In a closed system (one with no transfer of reactants to the outside world), the total amount of buffer present, B, is constant, i.e.

$$[HA] + [A^-] = B \tag{1.10}$$

where B is a constant. Thus, eqn (1.9) can be rewritten as

$$pH = pK + \log_{10}\frac{[A^-]}{B - [A^-]} \tag{1.11}$$

or

$$pH = pK + \log_{10}\frac{f}{1-f} \tag{1.12}$$

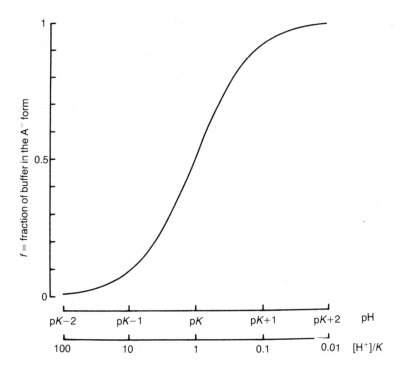

Fig. 1.2 The Henderson–Hasselbalch equation (equation (1.12) in the text). The fraction of a buffer solution in the basic form ($f = [A^-]/([A^-] + [HA]) = [A^-]/B$) as a function of pH. Note the two logarithmic scales for $[H^+]$ on the abscissa. The top scale is pH: when pH equals pK, $f = 1/2$. The bottom scale gives the corresponding values of $[H^+]$. Since the pH scale increases from left to right, the $[H^+]$ values increase from right to left.

where $f = [A^-]/B$ is the fraction of the buffer present in its basic (A^-) form. This equation is plotted in Figure 1.2. The pH equals the pK value for the buffer when $f = \frac{1}{2}$, i.e. when half the buffer is in the A^- form and half is in the HA form. Note that at pH values near pK (i.e. $[H^+]$ values near to K) the pH changes a relatively small amount as the fraction, f, of buffer in the A^- form is increased. In differential notation we can say that d(pH)/df is small. At pH values far from pK, the pH changes a lot as f is altered (d(pH)/df is large). When acid is added to a buffer system it tends to decrease the fraction of buffer in the A^- form, and increase the fraction in the HA form, because the added H^+ reacts with A^- to form HA ($H^+ + A^- \rightarrow HA$). Conversely, removal of H^+, e.g. by addition of OH^- to form H_2O, increases the fraction in the A^- form. The form of the graph in Figure 1.2 suggests that the pH change produced by adding or subtracting a given amount of H^+ (and thus changing f) will be large at pH values away from pK, but will be smaller at pH values near pK because the slope of the graph is larger (so a larger change of f has to occur to produce a given change of pH).

1.2.2 *Buffers work best for pH values near their pK value*
To prove the fact that buffers only work well at a pH near their pK value, we need to calculate how much the pH of a buffer solution changes when a certain amount of acid is added to the solution. Figure 1.2 does *not* tell us this because addition of a fixed amount of acid will not produce the same decrease in f at all values of pH. At very acid (low) pH values, the decrease in f produced when acid (H^+) is added will be very small, because f will already be close to zero. Conversely at high pH values (alkaline) almost all the buffer will be in the A^- form ($f = 1$), so adding H^+ will produce a large decrease in f. The following calculation derives a quantitative expression for the change of pH of a buffer solution produced when a small quantity of acid is added to it. The aim of this is to understand how the buffering power of a solution depends on the concentration and pK value of the buffer it contains.

The derivation starts by expressing eqn (1.6) in terms of the total concentration of buffer in the system, which is given as

$$B = [HA] + [A^-] \tag{1.10}$$

and the total concentration of protons in the system, which we can define as

$$C = [H^+] + [HA] \tag{1.13}$$

If we let $H = [H^+]$, eqns (1.10) and (1.13) can be rearranged to give

$$[HA] = C - H \tag{1.14}$$

and

$$[A^-] = H + B - C \tag{1.15}$$

Eqn (1.6) can thus be rewritten as

$$H = \frac{K(C - H)}{H + B - C} \tag{1.16}$$

or

$$H^2 + BH - CH = KC - KH \tag{1.17}$$

We now assume that $B \gg H$ and $B \gg K$, i.e. the concentration of buffer present is much higher than the free proton concentration and the value the free proton concentration would have when half the buffer present binds protons (when $H = K$). If these assumptions were not valid, the solution would not buffer very well at all. With these assumptions the terms H^2 and KH are much less than BH in eqn (1.17), which can thus be rewritten as

$$BH - CH = KC \tag{1.18}$$

or

$$C = \frac{BH}{K + H} \tag{1.19}$$

which relates the free proton concentration, H, to the total concentration of protons present, C.

By what small amount, dC, does the total amount of acid present have to be raised to increase H by the small amount dH? Differentiating eqn (1.19) with respect to H we get

$$\frac{dC}{dH} = \frac{BK}{(K + H)^2} \tag{1.20}$$

This equation can be inverted to get the change in H, dH, when C is increased by the small amount dC, as

$$\frac{dH}{dC} = \frac{(K+H)^2}{BK} \tag{1.21}$$

Actually we are interested in the **pH change** when acid is added, not the change in H. Now

$$\frac{d(\mathrm{pH})}{dC} = \frac{d(-\log_{10} H)}{dC} = \frac{-1}{H}\frac{dH}{dC}\frac{1}{\ln 10} \tag{1.22}$$

Note: $d(\log_{10} H)/dH = 1/(H \ln 10)$, where $\ln 10 = \log_e 10$; if you don't know how to differentiate logarithms see Bunday & Mulholland. Thus

$$d(pH)/dC = \frac{-(K+H)^2}{BKH \ln 10} = \frac{-(K+H)^2}{BKH(2.303)} \tag{1.23}$$

where 2.303 is $\ln 10$. This equation is written as a differential. For non-infinitesimal changes of pH and C we can rewrite it as

$$\Delta \mathrm{pH} = \frac{-(K+H)^2}{BKH\,2.303}\Delta C \tag{1.24}$$

where $\Delta \mathrm{pH}$ is the pH change produced when a concentration of acid ΔC is added.

Equation (1.24) is our final result. Notice the minus sign in this equation. This is present because when acid is added to the solution, increasing $[H^+]$, the pH goes **down**. There are two important points demonstrated by eqn (1.24). Firstly, the pH change produced when a given amount of acid is added to a buffer solution is inversely proportional to the total concentration of buffer in the solution, B. This is expected because the more buffer is present, the more protons will be able to bind to it. Secondly, the pH change occurring is a minimum when the pH equals the pK of the buffer (i.e. $[H^+] = K$). These points are demonstrated in Figure 1.3, where eqn (1.24) is plotted for the case where there is either 2 or 10 mmol$\cdot$l^{-1} of buffer present ($B = 2$ or 10 mmol$\cdot$l^{-1}) and where the amount of acid added to the solution is

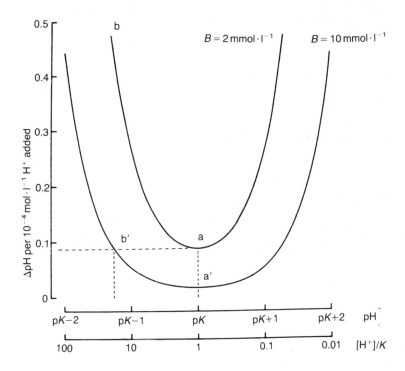

Fig. 1.3 Assessing the effectiveness of buffer solutions. The change in pH produced (ordinate) when $0.1\,\text{mmol}\cdot\text{l}^{-1}$ protons are added to a buffer solution containing 2 or $10\,\text{mmol}\cdot\text{l}^{-1}$ total buffer (equation (1.24)). The change in pH is inversely proportional to the buffering power of the solution. The buffering power is a maximum (i.e. ΔpH is at its lowest) when the pH equals the pK of the buffer (points a or a′). When the pH is more than one unit from the pK, the dilute buffer is not very effective (a large pH change is produced) (point b). Concentrated buffer can operate effectively over a wider pH range (compare ΔpH at point b′ for the more concentrated buffer and point b for the dilute buffer). This graph can be scaled to calculate the pH change produced for different amounts of added protons, ΔC, and different buffer concentrations, B. Equation (1.24) states that ΔpH is proportional to ΔC and inversely proportional to B.

$\Delta C = 10^{-4}\, \text{mol}\cdot\text{l}^{-1}$. If this amount of acid were added to an unbuffered neutral solution at pH 7 it would change the pH to the value 4 (pH $= -\log_{10} 10^{-4} = 4$), i.e. a change of 3 units.

Figure 1.3 shows that, as a rule of thumb, buffers will usefully minimise changes of pH when $[H^+]$ is added to, or removed from the system if the pH is within 1 unit of the pK value of the buffer, but outside this range they are much less effective. Note, however, the effect of buffer concentration: a solution containing 10 mmol $\cdot$ l^{-1} buffer, with the pH 1.3 units from its pK, buffers just as well as a solution containing only 2 mmol $\cdot$ l^{-1} buffer with the pH equal to the pK (compare points b' and a).

1.2.3 *Measuring buffering power in terms of pH or [H⁺] changes*

The idea of buffering being optimal around the point where pH $= pK$ depends crucially on the use of a logarithmic scale to measure $[H^+]$. What happens if we measure buffering power in terms of changes in $[H^+]$, rather than pH? We see from eqn (1.21) that the change, ΔH, of $[H^+]$ produced when ΔC of acid is added is given by

$$\Delta H = \frac{(K + H)^2}{BK} \Delta C \tag{1.25}$$

This is smallest when H is small, and gets larger as H gets bigger. In other words, if we measure buffering power in terms of minimising changes in $[H^+]$, then the buffering power is greatest at very alkaline pH (rather than when the pH equals the pK, as in Figure 1.3). This result is intuitively obvious: when H^+ is added, the amount removed (buffered) by reaction with A^- will be greatest when all of the buffer is in the A^- state (i.e. when H is very low to start with).

Why, then, do people think about buffering power in terms of **pH** changes? The answer is that, for most applications, it is not the absolute change in proton concentration, ΔH, that is important, but the fractional change relative to the initial value, $\Delta H/H$. In fact, the pH notation provides a measure of fractional changes in H: it can be shown that, for small changes in H,

$$\Delta pH = \frac{-\Delta H}{H} \frac{1}{\ln 10} = \frac{-\Delta H}{H} \frac{1}{2.303} \tag{1.26}$$

When protons are added to a buffer solution at very alkaline pH, although the change in free proton concentration, ΔH, is small, the change in pH is large because of the small value of H.

1.3 Buffer systems in the body

These can be divided up as follows:

In the blood:

   (i) In plasma: weak acids/bases on protein; bicarbonate; inorganic phosphate.

   (ii) In red cells: haemoglobin; bicarbonate; inorganic and organic phosphate.

In the extracellular fluid:

Like blood plasma but without protein. The volume of the extracellular fluid is nearly three times that of the blood, but has only a similar **total** buffering power to that of the blood because of the lack of protein (including haemoglobin).

In the intracellular fluid:

Protein; bicarbonate; phosphate (inorganic and organic).

In the urine:

Inorganic phosphate, ammonia, bicarbonate.

Let us see how the principles of buffer operation outlined above can be applied to these physiological buffers. We will start with inorganic phosphate buffer because it is the simplest. The aim of the following pages is to assess how well each of the buffer systems in the blood would reduce pH changes if it were the only buffer system operating. In the blood, of course, all the buffer systems operate together to minimise pH changes.

1.3.1 *Inorganic phosphate*

The reaction scheme for this buffer system is

$$H^+ + HPO_4^{2-} \rightleftharpoons H_2PO_4^- \qquad (1.27)$$

which has a pK value of 6.8. In normal blood, $[HPO_4^{2-}] = 1.04 \, \text{mmol} \cdot \text{l}^{-1}$ and $[H_2PO_4^-] = 0.26 \, \text{mmol} \cdot \text{l}^{-1}$. We can check for consistency with the Henderson–Hasselbalch equation (1.9): putting $[A^-] = 1.04 \, \text{mmol} \cdot \text{l}^{-1}$ and $[HA] = 0.26 \, \text{mmol} \cdot \text{l}^{-1}$, we find

$$pH = pK + \log_{10}([A^-]/[HA]) = 6.8 + \log_{10}(1.04/0.26) = 7.4$$

i.e. the pH of normal blood.

Now let us consider what happens if we add, say, $0.1\,\text{mmol}\cdot\text{l}^{-1}$ of H^+ (e.g. as the strong acid HCl) to a solution containing these concentrations of HPO_4^{2-} and $H_2PO_4^-$ (i.e. forgetting the other buffers in the body). In the absence of the phosphate buffer, the total concentration of H^+ present would be

$$\begin{aligned}
10^{-4}\,\text{mol}\cdot\text{l}^{-1} + 10^{-7.4}\,\text{mol}\cdot\text{l}^{-1} &= 100{,}000\,\text{nmol}\cdot\text{l}^{-1} + 40\,\text{nmol}\cdot\text{l}^{-1} \\
&= 100{,}040\,\text{nmol}\cdot\text{l}^{-1} \\
&= 0.10004\,\text{mmol}\cdot\text{l}^{-1}
\end{aligned}$$

This corresponds to a pH of 3.9998 – a rather acid pH which would cause death. The presence of the buffer completely changes the situation: when H^+ is added, the vast majority of it reacts with HPO_4^{2-} to form $H_2PO_4^-$. Thus, the concentration of HPO_4^{2-} will fall by approximately $0.1\,\text{mmol}\cdot\text{l}^{-1}$ to $0.94\,\text{mmol}\cdot\text{l}^{-1}$ and that of $H_2PO_4^-$ will rise by the same amount to $0.36\,\text{mmol}\cdot\text{l}^{-1}$. The new pH can be calculated from the Henderson–Hasselbalch equation (1.9) as

$$pH = 6.8 + \log_{10}(0.94/0.36) = 7.22$$

(an $[H^+]$ of $61\,\text{nmol}\cdot\text{l}^{-1}$). Thus, the presence of the buffer has reduced the pH decrease produced from 3.4 to 0.2 units!

Notice that, in this calculation, I assumed that **all** the added H^+ reacted with HPO_4^{2-}. Of course, not **all** of it does or there would be absolutely **no** change of pH! However, the fraction of the added H^+ that does not react is very small, $21\,\text{nmol}\cdot\text{l}^{-1}$ $(61 - 40\,\text{nmol}\cdot\text{l}^{-1})$ out of $100{,}000\,\text{nmol}\cdot\text{l}^{-1}$ in fact, and can be neglected in calculating the pH from the Henderson–Hasselbalch equation. This amounts to assuming, in advance, that the buffer is going to work well.

1.3.2 *The bicarbonate system (excluding CO_2 loss from the lungs)*
The reaction scheme for this system is

$$H^+ + HCO_3^- \rightleftharpoons H_2CO_3 \rightleftharpoons H_2O + CO_2 \qquad (1.28)$$

This is more complicated than the phosphate system because two reaction equilibria are involved. Furthermore, as we will see later, the system can be affected by loss of CO_2 from the lungs or HCO_3^- from the kidney. For the moment, though, let us ignore the fact that this loss of CO_2 or HCO_3^- can occur.

Let us start by considering the right-hand half of eqn (1.28). When CO_2 gas is in contact with water some of it dissolves, and a fraction of the dissolved CO_2 reacts with water:

$$CO_2 + H_2O \underset{k_2}{\overset{k_1}{\rightleftharpoons}} H_2CO_3 \tag{1.29}$$

This reaction proceeds slowly in simple solution, but the rate at which it reaches equilibrium is greatly increased in red blood cells by the enzyme carbonic anhydrase. From the law of mass action,

$$k_1[CO_2] = k_2[H_2CO_3] \tag{1.30}$$

in equilibrium. (Note that, by convention, the concentration of water is omitted from this equation because it is negligibly affected by this reaction, and is incorporated into the value of k_1.) Thus

$$\frac{[H_2CO_3]}{[CO_2]} = \frac{k_1}{k_2} = K \tag{1.31}$$

where $K \simeq 1/800 = 10^{-2.9}$. Thus, the ratio of H_2CO_3 to CO_2 dissolved in solution is very small. The commonly made statement that the majority of CO_2 dissolving becomes H_2CO_3 is true, but only because H_2CO_3 dissociates as follows to remove the end-product of reaction (1.29):

$$H_2CO_3 \underset{k_4}{\overset{k_3}{\rightleftharpoons}} H^+ + HCO_3^- \tag{1.32}$$

(the left-hand half of the reaction chain (1.28)). Applying the law of mass action to this, we get

$$\frac{[H^+][HCO_3^-]}{[H_2CO_3]} = \frac{k_3}{k_4} = K^1 \tag{1.33}$$

where K^1 is the equilibrium constant, and is about $10^{-3.2}\,mol \cdot l^{-1}$ (i.e. $pK^1 = 3.2$). At physiological (extracellular) pH (7.4), therefore, by rearranging eqn (1.33) we find

$$[HCO_3^-]/[H_2CO_3] = K^1/[H^+] = 10^{-3.2}/10^{-7.4}$$
$$= 10^{4.2}$$
$$\simeq 15,850 \qquad (1.34)$$

and we see that H_2CO_3 is a fairly strong acid because it is essentially completely dissociated.

We can obtain the relationship between pH and $[CO_2]$ by eliminating $[H_2CO_3]$ from eqns (1.31) and (1.33). Multiplying eqns (1.31) and (1.33) together we find

$$\frac{[H^+][HCO_3^-]}{[CO_2]} = KK^1 = K_{apparent} \qquad (1.35)$$

where $K_{apparent} = 10^{-2.9} \times 10^{-3.2}\,mol \cdot l^{-1} = 10^{-6.1}\,mol \cdot l^{-1}$. Now, by comparison with eqn (1.6) we see that this is the equation which would be obeyed if CO_2 reacted directly with water to give H^+ and HCO_3^- (without going through the H_2CO_3 stage), via a reaction with a dissociation constant $K_{apparent} = 10^{-6.1}\,mol \cdot l^{-1}$. Equation (1.35) can be rearranged, as for eqn (1.9), to give the Henderson–Hasselbalch equation for the bicarbonate buffer system:

$$pH = pK_{app} + \log_{10}\frac{[HCO_3^-]}{[CO_2]} \qquad (1.36)$$

with $pK_{app} = 6.1$.

The concentration, $[CO_2]$, of dissolved CO_2 is proportional to the partial pressure of CO_2 (PCO_2) in the gas with which the solution is in equilibrium. For arterial blood this PCO_2 is normally set by the CO_2 level in the alveoli at $5.33\,kPa$ (or $40\,mmHg$ in traditional units: $1\,mmHg = 133$ pascals $= 0.133\,kPa$). The constant relating $[CO_2]$ in $mmol \cdot l^{-1}$ to the PCO_2 is called the solubility constant. Its value is $0.225\,mmol \cdot l^{-1} \cdot kPa^{-1}$ (or $0.03\,mmol \cdot l^{-1} \cdot mmHg^{-1}$). Thus, the $[CO_2]$ is $0.225 \times 5.33 = 1.2\,mmol \cdot l^{-1}$. The value of $[HCO_3^-]$ in arterial blood is $23.94\,mmol \cdot l^{-1}$. (Check that, with these values, the pH you calculate from eqn (1.36) is indeed 7.4.) The concentration of H_2CO_3 in the blood is very small: re-arranging eqn (1.34) we find

$$[H_2CO_3] = [HCO_3^-]/15850 = 1.5 \, \mu mol \cdot l^{-1}$$

The effective pK of this buffer system, 6.1, is more than one pH unit from the normal pH in the plasma, and only slightly closer to the pH inside the red blood cell, so one would not expect it to be a very good buffer. Let us investigate this. Again, consider adding a concentration of $0.1 \, mmol \cdot l^{-1}$ extra H^+ to a solution containing the bicarbonate buffer at the concentration it has in the blood. Essentially all the added H^+ will react with HCO_3^-, producing CO_2. The $[HCO_3^-]$ will fall from 23.94 to $23.84 \, mmol \cdot l^{-1}$ and the $[CO_2]$ will rise to $1.3 \, mmol \cdot l^{-1}$ (ignoring removal of CO_2 by the lungs). Thus, the new pH is

$$pH = 6.1 + \log_{10}(23.84/1.3) = 7.36$$

i.e. the bicarbonate buffer has changed the pH reduction from the expected 3.4 units ($7.4 - 3.9998$) to 0.04 units ($7.4 - 7.36$).

How is it that the bicarbonate system can buffer relatively well even though its pK of 6.1 is so far from the physiological pH? Equation (1.24) and Figure 1.3 would suggest that the buffering should be poor. The reason for the good buffering is that the concentration of HCO_3^- is so high that, although the buffering power is relatively weak in the physiological pH range, it is still comparable with that of other buffers which have pK values nearer 7.4 but which are present at lower concentrations (compare the curves for $2 \, mmol \cdot l^{-1}$ and $10 \, mmol \cdot l^{-1}$ buffer in Figure 1.3). For example, if the bicarbonate buffer were present at a 10 times lower concentration (with $[HCO_3^-] = 2.4 \, mmol \cdot l^{-1}$ and $[CO_2] = 0.12 \, mmol \cdot l^{-1}$, comparable to the levels of the phosphate buffer considered above), the final pH expected in the example just considered would be 7.12 – a change of 0.28 rather than 0.04 units.

1.3.3 *The bicarbonate system (including CO_2 loss from the lungs)*
In the body the bicarbonate buffer works much better than is implied in the example above because, as we will see, changes in respiration result in the $[CO_2]$ in the blood being maintained

constant rather than rising when acid is added. Thus, the final pH reached in the previous example, if $[CO_2]$ were kept constant at $1.2 \, mmol \cdot l^{-1}$, would be $pH = 6.1 + \log_{10}(23.84/1.2) = 7.398$ i.e. a decrease of only 0.002 unit (as opposed to 0.04 unit expected in the absence of CO_2 being kept constant).

1.3.4 *Manipulations of the bicarbonate buffering system*

Quite apart from the quantitative aspects of buffering by the bicarbonate system, it is important to have an intuitive understanding of what the following manipulations do to the bicarbonate buffering system:

$$H^+ + HCO_3^- \rightleftharpoons H_2CO_3 \rightleftharpoons H_2O + CO_2 \qquad (1.28)$$

As discussed previously, if H^+ is added (for example from metabolism), it reacts with HCO_3^- to form H_2CO_3 and then CO_2 (i.e. the reactions proceed to the right). In the body this extra CO_2 will be lost by respiration.

What happens if HCO_3^- is added? This will react with H^+, driving the reaction to the right, and forming CO_2 which is lost. Thus, the pH rises (so addition of HCO_3^- can be used to treat acidosis).

What happens if CO_2 rises (for example, because respiration is insufficient)? The reaction proceeds to the left, and $[H^+]$ and $[HCO_3^-]$ rise. Conversely if $[CO_2]$ falls (e.g. through hyperventilation), the reaction proceeds to the right and $[H^+]$ and $[HCO_3^-]$ fall.

What happens if OH^- is added to the system? This will react with H^+, driving the reaction to the left, so CO_2 and H_2O are converted into H^+ and HCO_3^-, and $[HCO_3^-]$ rises.

1.3.5 *Buffering by proteins in general and haemoglobin in particular*

A protein like haemoglobin is a buffer because its molecule contains a number of acidic or basic groups with pK values near the physiological range. For example, carboxyl groups on amino acids dissociate like this:

$$R{-}COOH \rightleftharpoons R{-}COO^- + H^+ \qquad pK = 3\text{-}5$$

Terminal amino groups behave similarly:

$$R—NH_3^+ \rightleftharpoons R—NH_2 + H^+ \qquad\qquad pK \simeq 8$$

as does the sulfhydryl group of cysteine:

$$R—SH \rightleftharpoons R—S^- + H^+ \qquad\qquad pK \simeq 8.5$$

and the imidazole group of histidine:

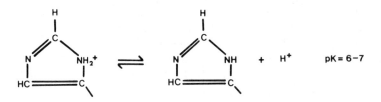

Imidazole groups are responsible for much of the buffering carried out by haemoglobin in the blood.

When the $[H^+]$ rises, these groups will bind protons, buffering the pH change that would otherwise occur. (Note that all these groups must be on the **outside** of the protein, accessible to the external solution, to act as buffers.) Although there is a relatively low concentration of haemoglobin in the blood ($150\,g \cdot l^{-1}$, with a molecular weight of 64458, giving a concentration of $2.33\,mmol \cdot l^{-1}$) it functions as a more effective buffer than, say, phosphate because it has more buffering groups per molecule. The various buffering groups have different pK values (range 6.5–7.8), so buffering by haemoglobin (and other proteins) cannot be characterised by a single Henderson–Hasselbalch equation as was done previously for simpler buffers. However, by titrating haemoglobin (Hb) solutions with acid, an empirical measurement of the buffering capacity has been obtained. For oxyhaemoglobin (HbO_2) in the physiological pH range, each $0.1\,mmol \cdot l^{-1}$ addition of H^+ to a solution containing $2.33\,mmol \cdot l^{-1}$ Hb (oxygenated, at $37\,°C$, in the presence of CO_2 at a partial pressure of $5.19\,kPa$ ($39\,mmHg$)) produces a pH change of 0.0015 unit. (This is calculated from Figure 7 of Davenport's book, *The ABC of acid–base chemistry*, cited in the section for further reading at the end of this chapter. Following common practice he gives the concentration of haemoglobin in milliequivalents, where one milliequivalent of HbO_2 relates to the O_2 part of the complex: as four O_2 molecules bind to each Hb molecule really, the buffering power per $mmol \cdot l^{-1}$ of Hb is actually four times that shown per milliequivalent in Davenport's graphs.)

1.4 Buffering power of blood components

We are now in a position to assess the relative importance of the different buffering components in the blood. The previous calculations have told us how much each buffer component would limit the pH change produced when a fixed amount of protons $(0.1 \, mmol \cdot l^{-1})$ is added to the blood. The results of the calculations are summarised in Table 1.2. Other blood proteins, and organic phosphate in red blood cells, make additional small contributions to buffering. In the short term, before the lungs can remove excess CO_2 (see below), the most important buffer is haemoglobin as it produces the smallest change in pH for a given amount of added acid. Next most important is bicarbonate, while phosphate makes a very small contribution. In the longer term, however, when the lungs have removed excess CO_2, the bicarbonate/CO_2 system makes nearly as large a contribution to minimising pH changes as does buffering by haemoglobin. (Of course this will not be true in cases of respiratory insufficiency, where it is a lack of removal of CO_2 by the lungs that is **causing** the pH change!)

Table 1.2. *Relative buffering power of blood components: the pH change produced when $0.1 \, mmol \cdot l^{-1} \, H^+$ is added to a solution containing each of these buffers alone with an initial pH of 7.4*

no buffer	3.4	units
phosphate	0.2	units
bicarbonate **without** removal of excess CO_2 ·	0.04	units
bicarbonate **with** removal of excess CO_2 by lungs	0.002	units
haemoglobin	0.0015	units

In calculating these pH changes, the concentration of each buffer is assumed to be its concentration in human blood.

In the blood, all these buffer systems are acting together to minimise pH changes, so the pH change produced is smaller than would occur if any one of the systems were present alone. Presence of more than one buffer system does not invalidate use of the Henderson–Hasselbalch equation to relate the concentration ratio of the buffer components to the pH. However, it complicates calculation of the change in pH when acid is added.

1.5 Further aspects of the bicarbonate buffer system

I have suggested above that the CO_2/HCO_3^- buffer system is important in controlling the pH of the body. The intimate dependence of this system on the CO_2 produced by metabolism makes it essential to understand the ways in which CO_2 is transported in the blood and how the lungs regulate the blood level of CO_2. This section is devoted to these topics.

1.5.1 *Transport of CO₂ in the blood*

When CO_2 enters the blood as a result of metabolism in the tissues it initially exists in simple solution. Some of it reacts with water to form carbonic acid (H_2CO_3) which dissociates to H^+ and HCO_3^-. The formation of carbonic acid is slow in plasma but, as CO_2 is relatively lipid soluble it rapidly enters red cells where the enzyme carbonic anhydrase speeds up the formation of carbonic acid by about 10^7 times. (Note that the formation of carbonic acid in the body may be limited by other factors such as the rate of diffusion of CO_2. Even so the rate of formation of carbonic acid in the body is about 13,000 times greater in the presence of carbonic anhydrase.) It is important to understand the fate of the H^+ and HCO_3^- thus generated. Since enzymes merely speed the rate at which reactions proceed towards equilibrium, the formation of H^+ and HCO_3^- would quickly stop if there were no removal of the end products of the reaction. In fact, the HCO_3^- formed leaves the red cell: as its concentration rises inside the cell, its electrochemical gradient drives it out of the cell. As HCO_3^- ions leave the cell, Cl^- ions enter the cell to maintain electroneutrality (this is the 'chloride shift' or 'Hamburger shift'). Consequently red cells in venous blood contain more Cl^- than red cells in arterial blood. These changes are illustrated in Figure 1.4.

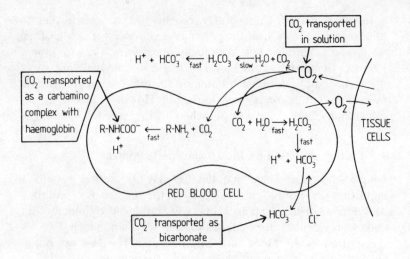

Fig. 1.4 The carriage of CO_2 in the blood. CO_2 leaving the tissues is carried in three ways in the blood: in simple solution, as a carbamino complex with haemoglobin in the red blood cells, and as HCO_3^- formed in red blood cells. The formation of HCO_3^- outside the red blood cells is slow, because of the absence of carbonic anhydrase. When the blood reaches the lungs, all the reactions shown in this figure are reversed (reverse the directions of the arrows, and replace the label 'tissue cells' by 'alveoli').

The reverse set of reactions occurs in the lungs: CO_2 leaves the plasma and enters the alveoli down its concentration gradient. This creates a concentration gradient promoting movement of CO_2 out of the red cell. The fall in $[CO_2]$ within the red cell results in HCO_3^- and H^+ in the red cell being converted into CO_2 and H_2O by carbonic anhydrase. As a result the $[HCO_3^-]$ falls inside the red cells, and HCO_3^- enters (in exchange for Cl^-) from the plasma.

Carbonic anhydrase in the red cells is responsible for the formation of the majority of the HCO_3^- in the plasma. Note, however, that it does not change the **absolute** level of HCO_3^- i.e. there is not **more** HCO_3^- than there could be in its absence. All carbonic anhydrase does is speed the interconversion of CO_2 and HCO_3^- so it can occur within the transit time of the blood through the capillaries of the peripheral tissues or alveoli.

What about the protons produced in the conversion of CO_2 to HCO_3^-? They are buffered by, for example, haemoglobin in the red cells.

In addition to the 80–90 per cent of CO_2 transported as HCO_3^- in the blood, and the 5 per cent or so that remains dissolved in solution as CO_2, there is another 5–15 per cent carried in direct combination with haemoglobin. This occurs because CO_2 can react with the N-terminal amino groups on all four chains of haemoglobin, to form carbamino compounds. This reaction

$$R—NH_2 + CO_2 \rightleftharpoons R—NHCOO^- + H^+ \qquad (1.37)$$

does not need a catalyst. (The amino groups on the β-chains of haemoglobin also bind 2,3-diphosphoglycerate–an organic phosphate modulator of the O_2 affinity of haemoglobin–and CO_2 competes with 2,3-diphosphoglycerate for the amino groups.) The reaction of CO_2 with haemoglobin has two important consequences. Firstly, it releases protons which have to be buffered by other sites on the haemoglobin molecule or by other buffers. Secondly, formation of carbamino compounds allosterically decreases the affinity of haemoglobin for O_2 (as does a rise in $[H^+]$ at constant $[CO_2]$). This potentiates the release of O_2 into the tissues where $[CO_2]$ is high (the Bohr effect). Conversely, binding of O_2 to haemoglobin reduces the affinity of its amino groups for CO_2 (the Haldane effect).

It appears, from (1.37) that CO_2 binding will result in haemoglobin releasing protons. This is true, but CO_2 binding is usually associated with O_2 unbinding, and the presence of O_2 bound to the iron groups of haemoglobin exerts an influence on the imidazole groups of histidines near the haem part of the molecule. As a result these groups have a more acidic pK when O_2 is bound, and a more alkali pK when O_2 is absent. Consequently, O_2 unbinding results in protons binding to these sites. In the physiological range the number of protons taken up in this way outweighs the number released by formation of carbamino compounds.

(These changes in the properties of haemoglobin were previously ignored, where the buffering power of oxyhaemoglobin maintained at constant $[CO_2]$ was given.)

1.5.2 *Control of [CO$_2$] by respiration*
In section 1.3.3 I explained that the efficiency of the bicarbonate
system as a buffer is greatly enhanced by the fact that, normally,
feedback systems exist to keep the arterial blood plasma [CO$_2$]
constant by altering the amount of CO$_2$ breathed out. Control of
the amount of CO$_2$ lost in this way is very important because of the
amount of CO$_2$ flux out through the lungs: about 330 litres are lost
per day (at rest). This is equivalent to 15 000 mmol of H$^+$ formed
from the reaction CO$_2$ + H$_2$O → H$_2$CO$_3$ → H$^+$ + HCO$_3^-$. For
comparison, the kidneys normally excrete about 50 mmol·day^{-1}
(maximum 600 mmol·day^{-1}) of H$^+$.

To exemplify the power of the lungs to regulate pH, suppose
that the rate of metabolic production of CO$_2$ is constant, and the
alveolar ventilation is altered from the value needed to maintain a
pH of 7.4. The CO$_2$ concentration in the arterial blood is roughly
inversely proportional to the alveolar ventilation. Halving the
ventilation doubles the [CO$_2$], and lowers the extracellular pH by
about 0.2 of a unit. In fact the ventilation can be reduced to almost
zero or increased to more than ten times normal, so the need for a
system to regulate respiration according to the [CO$_2$] is clear.

Changes in blood [CO$_2$] and pH modulate respiration by acting
on chemosensitive neurones in the medulla. It is believed the
primary effect on these neurones is due to H$^+$. However, CO$_2$ has
an indirect effect via its reaction with water to give H$^+$ (and
HCO$_3^-$). In fact, changes in arterial CO$_2$ have a bigger effect than
changes in arterial pH because CO$_2$ crosses the blood–brain
barrier much better than H$^+$ does. Thus, if arterial [CO$_2$]
increases, then [CO$_2$] diffuses into the medulla where it forms
carbonic acid and, thus, H$^+$ which stimulates the chemosensitive
neurones. These neurones then send a signal to the respiratory
control centres in the medulla, which in turn increase the rate and
depth of respiration. This increase in ventilation results in a loss of
more CO$_2$ from the body, and, thus, a lowering of arterial [CO$_2$]
and [H$^+$].

Alveolar ventilation is also controlled by the level of O$_2$ in
arterial blood. When the partial pressure of arterial O$_2$ falls below
about 11 kPa (80 mmHg), there is a steep increase in the impulse
activity from chemoreceptors in the carotid bodies (at the branch
of the carotid arteries) and aortic bodies (on the arch of the aorta)

which send impulses to the respiratory centres and, thus, increase the rate and depth of respiration. This effect is normally very small, however, because as soon as a low $[O_2]$ has increased respiration, CO_2 is lost so $[CO_2]$ and $[H^+]$ fall and, thus, respiration is decreased again by the chemosensitive areas in the medulla. It is only when $[CO_2]$ rises at the same time as $[O_2]$ falls that the O_2 chemoreceptors play a large role in regulating respiration. High $[CO_2]$ and $[H^+]$ also have an effect on the peripheral chemoreceptors, but this is small compared with their effects on the medullary chemoreceptors.

How is it that changes in blood $[CO_2]$ and $[H^+]$ can be corrected by changes in alveolar ventilation without drastically affecting the oxygen supply to the tissues? The answer is that the alveolar partial pressure of O_2 is normally sufficiently high to guarantee essentially 100 per cent saturation of haemoglobin. Even if alveolar ventilation is reduced to half normal (to compensate for a fall in $[CO_2]$ or $[H^+]$) haemoglobin still leaves the lungs 90 per cent saturated with O_2, because of the sigmoidal shape of the oxygen dissociation curve for haemoglobin. Thus, changes in respiration affect CO_2 exchange much more than O_2 exchange.

In addition to the control of respiration occurring via the medulla, there are also important local reflexes in the lungs, which act to maintain a balance between ventilation and blood perfusion in different areas of the lungs. For example, if an area of the lungs is poorly ventilated, so that the $[O_2]$ falls in the blood vessels from that area, then these blood vessels constrict, diverting blood to better ventilated areas. Conversely, if blood flow to part of the lungs is reduced, the lower CO_2 level in the alveoli of that area results in constriction of the bronchi to that area, shifting ventilation to better perfused areas of the lungs. These reflexes contribute to the maintainance of a normal arterial $[CO_2]$ and, hence, pH.

In exercise, O_2 consumption and CO_2 production can rise by twenty times, and alveolar ventilation increases to remove the excess CO_2 and avoid acidosis. However, only a small proportion of this increase in ventilation is due to the mechanisms described above. The increased ventilation is believed to result largely from information sent to the respiratory centres from the cerebral cortex, and joint, muscle and tendon receptors which report when the limbs are moving. The influence of the cerebral cortex explains why arterial [CO_2] can actually fall at the start of exercise – the brain anticipates the need for more alveolar ventilation than is actually necessary at first.

1.6 Renal regulation of acid–base balance

As previously mentioned, changes in respiration do not completely correct for alterations of blood pH. The kidneys can contribute to the regulation of pH by varying the amount of H^+ they excrete in the urine and the amount of HCO_3^- they reabsorb from the glomerular filtrate. The capacity of the kidneys to alter blood pH is much less than that of the lungs, but when given enough time to act (about three days) they can correct almost completely for deviations of blood pH from its normal value. Renal regulation of acid–base balance is dealt with in detail in Chapter 2 of this book.

1.7 Further reading

R. D. Bunday & H. Mulholland, *Pure mathematics for advanced level* (2nd edn). Chapter 12. Butterworths.

J. H. Comroe, *Physiology of respiration*. Yearbook Medical Publishers. Chapter 5 on control of respiration by CO_2; chapter 14 on O_2 and CO_2 transport in the blood; chapter 16 on the relationship between CO_2 and acid–base balance.

H. W. Davenport. *The ABC of acid–base chemistry*. Chicago University Press.

V. B. Mountcastle (1980). *Medical Physiology* (14th edn.) Mosby. Chapter 69 on transport of oxygen and carbon dioxide by the blood, and chapter 71 on chemical control of respiration at rest, by C. J. Lambertsen.

J. R. Robinson. *Fundamentals of acid–base regulation*. Blackwell Scientific.

L. Stryer. *Biochemistry*. W. H. Freeman. Chapter 4 on haemoglobin.

2

Renal control of acid–base balance

R. O. Law Department of Physiology, University of Leicester

2.1 Introduction

There are two closely inter-related aspects of acid–base balance which the kidney monitors and controls. The first involves elimination from the body of non-volatile acids; the second concerns the maintenance of concentrations of HCO_3^- sufficient to ensure adequate buffering of these acids prior to their excretion in the urine. (In this chapter the term 'secretion' is used to describe active and passive transport of solutes into tubular fluid and 'excretion', their eventual passage out of the kidney as ureteral urine.) Bicarbonate ion, HCO_3^-, is the body's most abundant buffer, about 5 mol being filtered daily by the kidneys (see Figure 2.1). Thus the kidneys have the dual task of regenerating plasma HCO_3^- (which has been used to buffer acid, see 1.3.2) and reabsorbing the filtered load of HCO_3^- which would otherwise be lost from the body. The renal mechanisms performing these functions play a major part in maintaining the pH of extracellular fluid within the range 7.36–7.44 (corresponding to a $[H^+]$ of 44–$36 \, \text{nmol} \cdot \text{l}^{-1}$; see Table 1.1).

Reabsorption of filtered HCO_3^- (see 2.3) occurs during conditions of normal acid–base balance and continues during imbalance states, although fractional reabsorption becomes depressed if the rate of tubular delivery increases significantly (see 2.3.2). (Fractional reabsorption is that fraction of the filtered load of a substance which is subsequently reabsorbed by the renal tubules; filtered load is the amount of a substance filtered in the glomerulus in unit time, e.g. $\text{mmol} \cdot \text{min}^{-1}$; rate of tubular delivery is the amount of a substance entering a given tubular segment in unit time, e.g. $\text{mmol} \cdot \text{min}^{-1}$.) Under basal conditions the body produces H^+ ions which are secreted into tubular fluid in exchange

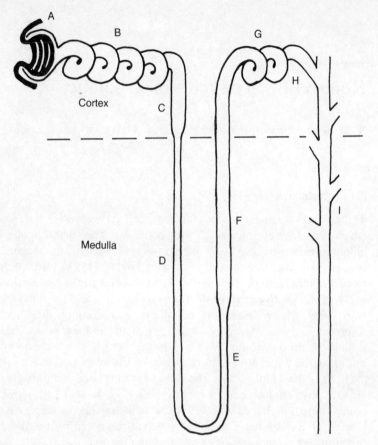

Fig. 2.1 Diagrammatic representation of a mammalian nephron showing the main segmental sub-divisions. A is the glomerulus (enclosed by Bowman's capsule), where passive filtration of plasma takes place. B and C are the convoluted and straight parts of the proximal tubule, where over 90 per cent filtered HCO_3^- is normally reabsorbed (see 2.3). Titratable acid secretion (see 2.4) and ammoniagenesis (see 2.4.1) also occur in these segments, although tubular fluid pH does not fall much below 7. D, E and F are, respectively, the descending, thin ascending and thick ascending limbs of Henle's loop. These segments normally play no part in acid–base regulation, although body fluid pH may be affected by the use of diuretic drugs acting on the thick ascending limb (see 2.8). G, the distal convoluted tubule, H, the collecting tubule, and I, the collecting duct, are collectively referred to as the distal nephron. Residual HCO_3^- reabsorption takes place, but their major role in acid–base control is secretion of high concentrations of titratable acid (see 2.4) and ammonia (see 2.4.1) during acidosis.

for reabsorbed Na^+ and HCO_3^-; thus urine is normally slightly acidic. At the same time, tubular cells regenerate HCO_3^- which has been destroyed by buffering H^+ in plasma.

It is the adaptability of these mechanisms which enables the healthy kidney to respond homeostatically to departures from normal acid–base balance. When the pH of body fluids falls (acidosis) or rises (alkalosis) alterations in the rates of H^+ secretion and HCO_3^- regeneration occur which tend to return plasma pH and HCO_3^- to normal levels. (Although under certain circumstances acid–base imbalance can be localised to a specific fluid compartment, see, for example, 2.6, it is often manifest uniformly throughout the body fluids; plasma is commonly taken as the reference fluid since it is easily sampled.) For example, increased production of non-CO_2 acid (metabolic acidosis) resulting in an increase in intracellular H^+, leads to an increase in the acidity of tubular fluid by activation of a $Na^+–H^+$ exchange (see 2.3.3.1). Depleted plasma HCO_3^- is also restored (see 2.4) and there is enhanced renal ammoniagenesis (see 2.4.1). An increase in the filtered load of HCO_3^- due to raised plasma $[HCO_3^-]$ (metabolic alkalosis) is accompanied, as previously mentioned, by depressed fractional tubular reabsorption of HCO_3^-. Until plasma composition has been restored to normal, the medullary chemoreceptors trigger compensation, in accordance with the Henderson–Hasselbalch equation, by adjusting the rate of alveolar CO_2 elimination so that arterial plasma PCO_2 falls (in metabolic acidosis) or increases (in metabolic alkalosis) (see Chapter 1). Acidosis due to alveolar CO_2 retention (with a rise in arterial PCO_2) increases the rate of tubular fluid acidification, the excess CO_2 being converted by the kidney to H^+ (secreted) and HCO_3^-, which leads to a compensatory rise in plasma $[HCO_3^-]$: converse processes operate during respiratory alkalosis. Renal compensation of respiratory acid–base balance is considered in section 2.5. Note that, with a single exception (see 2.4.2), disturbances of acid–base balance are not of renal origin.

2.2 The source of excreted hydrogen ions

H^+ ions are a normal end product from the catabolism of a mixed diet; alkaline substances are not directly formed by the body in significant amounts. Unlike their conjugate anions, extracellular H^+ ions are almost completely buffered, e.g. by HCO_3^-, HPO_4^{2-} and plasma proteins (see Chapter 1). At pH 7.4, $[H^+]$ in plasma is approximately $40\,nmol \cdot l^{-1}$. However, even during normal acid–base balance 50–80 mmol H^+ are eliminated daily in urine (as titratable acid and NH_4^+, see 2.4). This large urinary H^+ load (by comparison with plasma) cannot be accounted for simply by the urinary concentrating process; urinary acidification must reflect the ability of renal tubular cells to produce and secrete H^+. This fundamental aspect of renal function has long been recognised. Renal cells secrete H^+ at a rate which is approximately proportional to their H^+ content, and should the secretory mechanism become impaired a condition known as renal tubular acidosis will result (see 2.4.2).

2.2.1 *Urinary pH*
The pH of urine lies between 4.5 and 8.2, and for reasons already stated it is normally more acidic than plasma. It is governed principally by the difference between the rate of glomerular filtration of HCO_3^- and the rate of tubular secretion of H^+. As already mentioned (see 2.1) the latter is influenced both by arterial plasma PCO_2 and by intracellular pH in the renal tubules. However, it should be stressed that some areas of uncertainty in our understanding of the control of H^+ secretion stem from the impracticability of studying several controlling factors in isolation, e.g. arterial and tubular fluid PCO_2, $[HCO_3^-]$ and pH. Some of our current knowledge derives from experiments on analogous but more easily manipulated structures such as the isolated turtle bladder. Its 'tight' epithelium (one with cells in close contact and so able to maintain a steep electrochemical gradient) has some characteristics resembling those of the mammalian distal tubule.

In order to achieve a urinary pH as low as 4.5, e.g. during severe metabolic acidosis, at least some part of the nephron must be capable of secreting H^+ against a concentration gradient of nearly 1000:1. The precise magnitude of this gradient will partly depend on renal intracellular pH. In the mammalian proximal tubule this probably does not fall below about pH 7.2, due to the presence of intracellular buffers. However, it is important to bear in mind that this figure represents a **concentration**, and does not directly reflect the **amount** of H^+ ions available for secretion or the cell's secretory activity. Little is known about intracellular pH in the distal nephron (i.e. the distal tubule, collecting tubule and collecting duct) where the highest levels of tubular acidification occur (see 2.3.1 and 2.4).

2.3 Reabsorption of filtered bicarbonate

2.3.1 *Basic cellular mechanisms*
In order to prevent depletion of the body's principle extracellular buffer, filtered HCO_3^- is normally completely reabsorbed along the nephron (leading to the production of neutral or acidic urine). The reabsorptive process is critically dependent upon the ability of tubular cells to produce and secrete H^+ ions. During both reabsorption and restoration of HCO_3^- the two ion species are exchanged on a 1:1 basis, i.e. the rate of tubular H^+ secretion can be inferred from the rate of plasma alkalinisation and *vice versa*.

Figure 2.2*a* summarises the process of HCO_3^- reabsorption as it is most frequently depicted in textbooks. Intracellular H^+ is derived from the splitting of H_2CO_3, which is formed from the reaction of cell water with the CO_2 which has entered the cell down a chemical concentration gradient following titration of filtered HCO_3^- by secreted H^+. This is a normal process, in the sense that it occurs whether or not there has been any change in extracellular pH. Although it involves H^+ secretion it is quite distinct from the process of tubular acidification (see 2.4), the secreted H^+ being excreted as water. It is influenced by body acid–base balance only in so far as this affects the length of the nephron over which reabsorption takes place. Under normal conditions a small fraction of filtered HCO_3^- passes out of the proximal tubule. The concentration of HCO_3^- in late proximal tubular fluid is normally about $5-8 \, mmol \cdot l^{-1}$, and if it is assumed that the concentration in glomerular filtrate is $25 \, mmol \cdot l^{-1}$ and that 75 per cent volume reabsorption occurs in the proximal tubule, it can readily be calculated that some 5–8 per cent of the filtered load reaches the distal tubule (assuming negligible destruction in Henle's loop), where it is reabsorbed by mechanisms analogous to those in Figure 2.2. In acute metabolic acidosis, however, reabsorption is complete in the proximal

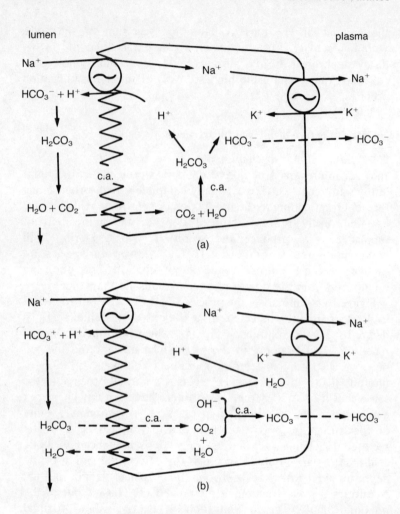

Fig. 2.2 The reabsorption of filtered HCO_3^- by proximal tubular cells. (a) shows the mechanism as it is usually envisaged although, as described in the accompanying text, there are several areas of uncertainty. These include the tightness of the Na^+–H^+ antiport, the mode of peritubular HCO_3^- extrusion, the source of the cellular H^+ and the identity of the molecular species crossing the luminal brush border. Alternative possibilities for the latter two are incorporated in (b). Active and passive membrane transport processes are indicated by solid and dashed lines respectively. c.a. = carbonic anhydrase.

tubule: tubular fluid is already somewhat acidified (see 2.4) by the time it leaves this segment (although the pH does not fall far below 7.0). Conversely, during alkalosis complete HCO_3^- reabsorption may not occur at all, with the result that HCO_3^- is spilled into an alkaline urine.

An alternative possibility, shown in Figure 2.2*b*, is that H^+ ions are derived from H atoms formed from the metabolic splitting of water and subsequently oxidised by Fe^{3+} in the cytochrome system, with the ultimate production of intracellular OH^- ions. The operation of this redox pump may be represented thus

$$4Fe^{3+} + 4H \rightleftharpoons 4Fe^{2+} + 4H^+ \tag{2.1}$$

$$4Fe^{2+} + O_2 + H_2O \rightleftharpoons 4Fe^{3+} + 4OH^- \tag{2.2}$$

CO_2 entering the cell from luminal fluid is hydroxylated by the residual OH^-, a reaction which may be catalysed by cytosolic carbonic anhydrase (see 2.3.1.1). This mechanism could raise the intracellular electrochemical potential of H^+ to a very high level; higher, indeed, than would be required even for the purpose of maximum urinary acidification.

2.3.1.1 *Renal carbonic anhydrase.* Both the breakdown of tubular H_2CO_3 in the region of the luminal membrane (the brush border) and its subsequent intracellular reformation (Figure 2.2*a*) are facilitated by the presence of the enzyme carbonic anhydrase, as also is the hydroxylation of CO_2 (Figure 2.2*b*). This zinc metalloenzyme greatly accelerates the attainment of equilibrium in step (i) of the reaction

$$CO_2 + H_2O \overset{(i)}{\rightleftharpoons} H_2CO_3 \overset{(ii)}{\rightleftharpoons} H^+ + HCO_3^- \tag{2.3}$$

It is important to remember that, like all organic catalysts, the enzyme facilitates both the forward and the backward reaction (hence its alternative name carbonate hydrolase), and that the reaction can occur, although much more slowly, in the absence of the enzyme. Step (ii) is inherently rapid. Immunochemical and histochemical techniques have shown that a small but important

fraction of cortical carbonic anhydrase (<5 per cent) is located in
the brush border of proximal tubular cells where it is presumed to
be in functional contact with the tubular fluid. Luminal carbonic
anhydrase is not found in the distal tubule. The enzyme is
inhibited by certain drugs, e.g. acetazolamide, and much of our
knowledge of the functional importance of renal carbonic
anhydrase comes from studying the consequences of its inhibition.
Luminal and cytosolic carbonic anhydrases can be selectively
inhibited (see 2.3.1.2): the former is much the more acetazola-
mide-resistant. In addition to that in the cortex, carbonic anhydrase is found in cells in the thick ascending limb of Henle's loop
(the diluting segment); its function is not certain but it is probably
not directly related to acid–base control.

2.3.1.2 *Disequilibrium pH*. An important aspect of the reaction
between secreted H^+ and filtered HCO_3^- is the extent (if any) to
which tubular fluid pH is lowered by the transient presence of
H_2CO_3, since this will directly affect the concentration gradient
against which H^+ must be secreted. Until H_2CO_3 has dissociated
into CO_2 and water tubular acidity will be greater than that
predicted by the Henderson–Hasselbalch equation on the assumption of equilibrium with peritubular CO_2. (This equilibrium is
never in fact attained *in vivo*, since tubular PCO_2 remains higher
than arterial PCO_2.) This discrepancy is known as an **acidic
disequilibrium pH**, and can be defined as the quantitative
difference between the observed pH and the calculated pH. The
extent of the disequilibrium (if any) will depend mainly upon the
rate of dissociation of the H_2CO_3 and, hence, upon the nephron
segment studied. Thus, no disequilibrium pH can normally be
recorded in the proximal tubule, where luminal carbonic anhydrase is present. However, the presence of residual HCO_3^- in
the distal tubule, where there is no luminal enzyme, can lead to a
disequilibrium pH of nearly one pH unit, hence to a near ten-fold
increase in the gradient against which H^+ must be secreted. In
metabolic acidosis, when HCO_3^- reabsorption is almost or wholly
complete in the proximal tubule, distal disequilibrium is reduced
or abolished, thus facilitating homeostatic H^+ secretion. The
significance of luminal carbonic anhydrase in relation to acidic
disequilibrium pH is clearly demonstrated by the observation that

selective inhibition of this enzyme causes a marked decrease in HCO_3^- reabsorption, accompanied by disequilibrium pH, whereas selective inhibition of the cytosolic enzyme causes comparable reduction of HCO_3^- reabsorption without disequilibrium. (Although disequilibrium pH is normally ascribed to undissociated H_2CO_3, it is clear that a small contribution must be due to the tubular fluid/plasma PCO_2 imbalance referred to previously.)

In the converse situation, active removal of tubular HCO_3^- in the presence of non-HCO_3^- buffers shifts the equilibrium in eqn (2.3) to the right. Hence, an **alkaline disequilibrium pH** will be established, since the H_2CO_3 term in the Henderson–Hasselbalch equation will be reduced.

2.3.2 *Transport of bicarbonate*

HCO_3^- is a relatively large anion, and cell membranes might be assumed to be less permeable to it than to smaller anions such as Cl^-. It should be noted that neither of the pathways in Figure 2.2 requires unchanged HCO_3^- to cross the luminal membrane. It is possible that carbonic anhydrase facilitates luminal CO_2 transport by transiently hydrating it to H_2CO_3, which is even more lipid soluble than CO_2 itself; alternatively, it may be the case that H_2CO_3 formed from the reaction between H^+ and luminal HCO_3^- is itself the transported species. The latter possibility is represented in Figure 2.2*b*.

It should be mentioned that limited HCO_3^- permeability of cell membranes in the diluting segment may impair hyperosmotic Na^+ reabsorption when HCO_3^- delivery from the proximal tubule is elevated; this could account for the concentrating and diluting defects which characterise metabolic alkalosis.

As with luminal entry, there is no certainty as to the process of peritubular HCO_3^- extrusion. The peritubular membrane may have an abnormally high HCO_3^- permeability; alternatively there may again be a role for carbonic anhydrase in this process. Extrusion is sensitive to certain stilbenesulphonic acid derivatives known to inhibit anion exchange processes, suggesting that a HCO_3^- for Cl^- antiport may operate. A further possibility is that OH^- (e.g. as produced in Figure 2.2*b*) may be the extruded species, reconversion to HCO_3^- being due to extracellular CO_2. Whatever the nature of the extruded anion it is likely to be influenced by the activity of the peritubular electrogenic Na^+–K^+ antiport (the Na^+ pump).

Whatever the nature of the transport phenomena at the level of cell membranes it is clear that under normal conditions they are adequate to permit proximal reabsorption of over 90 per cent filtered HCO_3^- (see 2.3.1), with distal reabsorption of the remainder. Fractional reabsorption (i.e. that proportion of filtered HCO_3^- which is reabsorbed) is influenced by plasma HCO_3^- concentration. In most mammals this is 24–26 mmol·l^{-1}. Under conditions of normal acid–base balance, when no HCO_3^- appears in urine (i.e. fractional reabsorption is 100 per cent), this implies a reabsorptive rate of 3–4 mmol·min^{-1}. If the kidneys are required to reabsorb HCO_3^- at a higher rate, e.g. due to raised plasma and filtrate HCO_3^- concentration during metabolic alkalosis, or to increase glomerular filtration rate, fractional reabsorption becomes depressed and an alkaline urine is excreted. The highest plasma HCO_3^- concentration which is compatible with 100 per cent fractional reabsorption (assuming normal glomerular filtration rate) is sometimes referred to as the 'renal HCO_3^- threshold': it approximates to normal plasma HCO_3^- concentration, although its precise value will depend upon the rates of tubular H^+ secretion and Na^+ reabsorption (Figure 2.2). Despite the fall in fractional reabsorption, however, there appears to be no ceiling on the **absolute** reabsorptive capacity of the nephron. The ease with which this can be demonstrated depends upon experimental conditions, in particular whether or not steps are taken to control the body's extracellular fluid volume. If this is allowed to increase, fractional reabsorption of filtered Na^+ and its conjugate anions (Cl^- and HCO_3^-) will be depressed by a variety of intrarenal and extrarenal natriuretic responses and an apparent absorptive ceiling for HCO_3^- will be approached asymptotically.

2.3.2.1 *Direct reabsorption of bicarbonate.* It is likely that a significant fraction of filtered HCO_3^- is reabsorbed as the unchanged anion by a mechanism which is neither carbonic anhydrase-dependent nor directly linked to H^+ secretion. As has already been pointed out, step (i) in equation (2.3) and, hence, the reactions summarised in Figure 2.2, can still proceed when carbonic anhydrase is inhibited, albeit slowly. (Experimental data relating to this are sometimes difficult to interpret since the degree of carbonic anhydrase inhibition is not always certain.) In addition to this there is evidence of direct HCO_3^- reabsorption. Little is known of the mechanism or mechanisms involved, but it appears to be inhibited by maleate, which acts additively with acetazolamide (thus providing good evidence for two distinct reabsorptive processes) and by Li^+. According to one estimate up to 50 per cent of filtered HCO_3^- may be directly reabsorbed. It is interesting to note that dependence of HCO_3^- reabsorption upon carbonic anhydrase in mammals diminishes during acid–base disturbances (metabolic and respiratory acidosis and metabolic alkalosis), which suggests a reversion to the mode of reabsorption observed in certain relatively primitive vertebrates. In the case of alkalosis this independence may be simply the result of an elevated HCO_3^- concentration gradient between luminal and tubular fluids, but under acidotic conditions a direct reabsorptive mechanism seems probable.

Note that direct movement of HCO_3^- across the luminal brush border is not incompatible with simultaneous addition of H^+ to tubular fluid: this could occur if the HCO_3^- were derived not from filtrate but from the reaction between water and metabolic CO_2 from renal cells.

2.3.3 *Coupled bicarbonate and sodium reabsorption*

As shown in Figure 2.2, the presence of filtered Na^+ ions is essential for HCO_3^- reabsorption and for H^+ secretion. Na^+–H^+ exchange is shown in a $1:1$ basis (electroneutral) but it should be stressed that only a fraction of Na^+ reabsorption is dependent on this exchange. Figure 2.2 considers only those Na^+ ions which are covered by HCO_3^-; about 80 per cent of filtered Na^+ is covered by Cl^- and reabsorption of this fraction occurs by other processes, active and passive, which lie outside the scope of this book.

2.3.3.1 *The sodium-hydrogen ion antiport.*

Several observations suggest, and recent evidence confirms, the existence of a Na^+–H^+ antiport on the luminal membrane of renal tubular cells. The necessity for active H^+ pumping can be inferred mainly from events in the distal nephron, where even the highest transepithelial electrical potential difference (lumen $-50\,mV$ with respect to peritubular fluid) would be inadequate to account for the observed rates of tubular acidification (see 2.4). Adrenalectomy (which causes impaired Na^+ reabsorption in the distal nephron) reduces H^+ secretion. (These effects may be due not only to lack of aldosterone but also to lack of glucocorticoids, which have recently been shown to accelerate the Na^+–H^+ antiport in renal brush border membrane vesicles.) The latter finding confirms the existence of a proximal tubular antiport, which might otherwise be questioned in view of the negligible acidification which normally takes place in this segment. The presence of tubular HCO_3^- and an active Na^+ pump, for example, might be regarded as sufficient to drive H^+ secretion, and it is indeed the case that ouabain (a specific inhibitor of the Na^+ pump) depresses by up to 80 per cent both H^+ secretion and HCO_3^- reabsorption in isolated proximal tubules from the rabbit (but not the ouabain-resistant rat). Some active H^+ secretion, however, must occur in this segment in order to account for the small but discernible proximal acidification which occurs in metabolic acidosis. As to its dependence upon Na^+, it has proved possible in the doubly-perfused rat kidney tubule largely to uncouple H^+ and Na^+ exchange by suitable manipulation of tubular buffers; a far tighter coupling occurs in the rabbit. (These observations highlight the difficulties encountered by investigators due to species differences. Although we may assume that man conforms to the overall pattern observed in laboratory animals, we know little of human-specific events at cellular level.) A Na^+–H^+ antiport has now been identified in the proximal brush border of both species. In addition to the effect of glucocorticoids mentioned previously, it is sensitive to the drug amiloride, although considerably higher concentrations are needed than for amiloride's better characterised action of blocking Na^+ entry across the luminal membrane of tight epithelia such as the distal tubule.

As already pointed out, there is good reason to believe in the existence of a Na^+–H^+ antiport, presumably tightly coupled, in the distal and collecting tubules and the collecting duct, although these segments are more difficult to examine experimentally. In both sites, enhanced tubular acidification during metabolic acidosis may be due, at least in part, to a direct effect of intracellular pH on antiport activity. It is to this aspect of renal acid–base control that this chapter now turns.

2.4 Urinary acidification and the restoration of depleted bicarbonate

So far this chapter has been chiefly concerned with the reabsorption of filtered HCO_3^-, a process which, while it is influenced by body acid–base status (notably in respect of the length of nephron over which reabsorption takes place), is not a functional response to conditions of imbalance and does not correct them. The remission of acidosis, and the restoration of normal plasma HCO_3^- concentration, requires the secretion of H^+ not as water (Figure 2.2) but as free and buffered protons.

Under normal conditions some 20–30 mmol of titratable acid are excreted daily in human urine. This derives mainly from the catabolism of sulphur-containing proteins (to give sulphuric acid) and phosphorus-containing compounds such as phospholipids (to give phosphoric acid). During their passage from the site of production to the kidneys these acids are buffered by reaction with plasma HCO_3^-. For example

$$H_2SO_4 + 2NaHCO_3 \rightleftharpoons Na_2SO_4 + 2H_2O + 2CO_2 \qquad (2.4)$$

The resultant fall in plasma pH (a) stimulates the medullary chemoreceptors, leading to pulmonary elimination of excess CO_2 and a compensatory fall in plasma PCO_2, and (b) increases activity of the renal tubular Na^+-H^+ antiport, via secondary reduction in intracellular pH, leading to increased secretion of titratable acid. In severe acidosis the secretory level may rise to as much as $200\,mmol \cdot day^{-1}$, e.g. in untreated diabetes mellitus (aceto-acetic acid and β-hydroxybutyric acid), salicylate intoxication or lactate acidosis. Under both normal and acidotic conditions the elimination of H^+ is directly linked to the reconstitution of the HCO_3^- which has been destroyed in eqn (2.4), and it is necessary clearly to distinguish this restorative process from the reabsorption described in section 2.3. The relevant events are shown in Figure 2.3. The bulk of the secreted H^+ is buffered by filtered HPO_4^{2-} (a smaller fraction is buffered by creatinine). The resultant $H_2PO_4^-$ is weakly acidic:

$$H_2PO_4^- \rightleftharpoons H^+ + HPO_4^{2-} \qquad (2.5)$$

However, since the pK of this reaction is greater than 4.5 (i.e. the limiting pH of urine), the anion can be excreted whereas strong

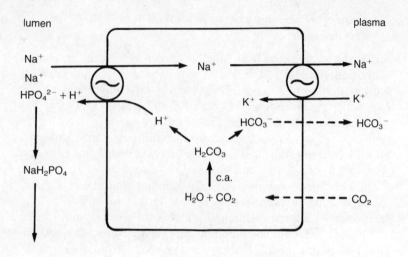

Fig. 2.3 Secretion of titratable acid in the form of NaH_2PO_4.

acids ($pK < 4.5$) cannot. At pH 4.5 the equilibrium in eqn (2.5) is almost completely to the left. The reactions in Figure 2.3 can occur both proximally and distally, although far higher concentrations of acid are encountered in the distal nephron. The exact amount of titratable acid in urine can be estimated by back-titrating to plasma pH with NaOH:

$$NaOH + NaH_2PO_4 \rightleftharpoons Na_2HPO_4 + H_2O \qquad (2.6)$$

Note the dependence of the mechanism upon cytosolic carbonic anhydrase, also that the events in Figure 2.3 do not represent the only method of restoring plasma HCO_3^-, since non-HCO_3^- buffers in plasma (represented as Buf^-) also participate:

$$H_2O + CO_2 + Buf^- \rightleftharpoons HBuf + HCO_3^- \qquad (2.7)$$

Paradoxically, enhanced alveolar elimination of the CO_2 produced in eqn (2.4) during the respiratory compensation of metabolic acidosis somewhat reduces the extent to which renal H^+ secretion would otherwise be elevated, but the concomitant reduction in arterial PCO_2 has the effect of moderating the depression of plasma pH.

The rate at which H^+ can be eliminated as titratable acid depends upon the availability of filtered HPO_4^{2-} which, in turn, is determined both by plasma concentration and by glomerular filtration rate. The filtered load, normally approximately $100\,\mu mol \cdot min^{-1}$, is inadequate to buffer all the H^+ which must be secreted during severe prolonged acidosis. Therefore, a second mechanism for buffering tubular H^+ must be available.

2.4.1 *Renal ammoniagenesis*
This mechanism involves the buffering of H^+ as the very weak conjugate acid NH_4^+ and depends upon the ability of the kidney to synthesise and secrete NH_3. This occurs both proximally and, at much higher concentrations, distally. The free base exists in equilibrium with NH_4^+:

$$NH_4^+ \rightleftharpoons H^+ + NH_3 \qquad (2.8)$$

The pK of this reaction in mammalian plasma is about 9.2; thus, at equilibrium and at physiological pH the reaction will be strongly to the left: only just over 1 per cent free base will be present. However, since this is very much more lipid-soluble than NH_4^+ it is able readily to diffuse into the tubular fluid where it is re-converted to NH_4^+ by secreted H^+. This is shown in Figure 2.4. The charged form cannot readily back-diffuse into tubular cells, so provided there is continuous tubular fluid flow a secretory concentration gradient for NH_3 will be maintained. The steepness of this gradient is determined principally by tubular pH. Thus, at pH 6 the tubular $NH_4^+ : NH_3$ ratio at equilibrium will be $10^3 : 1$, and a potential ten-fold secretory gradient will exist. At pH 5 the gradient will be 100-fold. In a free-flowing tubule equilibrium will never be achieved. The slower the flow the more nearly the expected $NH_4^+ : NH_3$ **ratio** will be approached, but this does not mean that the secretory **gradient** will become more favourable, since the diffusible species (NH_3) will tend to equilibrate across the luminal membrane, with tubular NH_4^+ concentration rising to maintain the ratio. This method of passive secretion of weak bases into acidic tubular fluid (and of weak acids into alkaline fluid) is known as ionic or diffusion trapping, and the pH and rate of formation of urine may be significant in determining the rate of elimination of weakly basic (e.g. quinine) or acidic (e.g. phenobar-

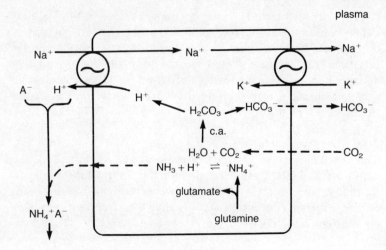

Fig. 2.4 Renal production and secretion of ammonia.

bitone) drugs from the body. Although NH_3 can also diffuse across the peritubular membrane its tendency to do so will be constrained by the pH difference between renal interstitial and tubular fluids, which will normally, and particularly during acidosis, favour tubular secretion due to far more efficient ionic trapping.

Ammoniagenesis also relieves the body of the need to waste osmotically valuable Na^+ as the covering cation for the organic (e.g. aceto-acetate) and inorganic (e.g. SO_4^{2+}) anions excreted during acidosis. For example, the Na_2SO_4 produced in eqn (2.4) will be recovered in the renal tubules:

$$Na_2SO_4 + 2H^+ + 2NH_3 \rightleftharpoons (NH_4)_2SO_4 \text{ (excreted)} + 2Na^+ \text{ (reabsorbed)} \qquad (2.9)$$

Some 30–50 mmol H^+ are normally secreted daily as NH_4^+. Thus, the sum of H^+ ions secreted as titratable acid plus NH_4^+ is 50–80 mmol · day^{-1}, although during prolonged metabolic acidosis this figure can reach 600 mmol as increased NH_3 production accompanies increased secretion of $H_2PO_4^-$ (see 2.4). (For comparison it is worth noting that the lungs normally eliminate some 15,000 mmol of volatile acid per day in the form of CO_2!)

The source of renal NH_3 was the subject of extensive studies in dogs by R. F. Pitts and his colleagues during the 1960s (see 2.9). Fifty per cent or more of secreted NH_3 is derived from glutamine, which is converted to glutamic acid by the enzyme glutaminase, the glutamic acid then being deaminated to α-ketoglutaric acid by glutamate dehydrogenase. Both steps in this reaction yield one molecule of NH_3. As much as one third of secreted NH_3 may be extracted from arterial plasma (down a chemical concentration gradient and with the assistance of ionic trapping). This NH_3 is probably mainly of renal origin, having previously left the kidney via the venous drainage.

For reasons which are not clearly understood, ammoniagenesis during metabolic acidosis may take as long as a week to attain maximum levels. In the rat, at least, the onset of metabolic acidosis may be accompanied by a transient **inhibition** of ammoniagenesis (while metabolic alkalosis temporarily enhances it). There are, presumably, certain relatively slow adaptive alterations in the ammoniagenetic pathways during chronic acidosis; possibilities include an increased rate of mitochondrial glutamine transport and a reduction of product-inhibition of glutaminase due to an increased rate of glutamate deamination. As for the initial stimulus to such changes, this is probably not simply the fall in extracellular pH, since were this the case respiratory acidosis should cause ammoniagenesis; there is little convincing evidence that this occurs during chronic hypercapnia, and it has been shown in the rat that respiratory acidosis does not enhance renal glutaminase activity. The stimulus may be increased intracellular H^+ content, or decreased K^+ content (see 2.6). There is evidence that secretion of glucocorticoids, which are known to stimulate ammoniagenesis, increases during metabolic acidosis.

2.4.2 *Renal tubular acidosis*
In acute or advanced chronic renal failure both glomerular filtration (i.e. the supply of tubular HPO_4^{2-}) and ammoniagenesis are depressed, and the kidney loses its ability to secrete adequate amounts of H^+. The condition of renal tubular acidosis results. In the case of ammoniagenesis this represents a dysfunction of the renal cells themselves, whereas in generalised metabolic acidosis there is normally no impairment of cellular function.

2.5 Renal compensation of respiratory acid–base disturbances

Compensatory processes, both renal and respiratory, imply the reduction of extracellular pH changes which otherwise accompany acid–base disturbances; they do not correct the underlying imbalance, only one of its manifestations. Thus, for example, enhanced pulmonary ventilation can act as a temporary partial compensation for the over-production of fixed acids by shifting the equilibrium in eqn (2.4) to the right, but a longer-term adaptive renal process, secretion of titratable acid and ammonia and the restoration of depleted plasma HCO_3^-, are needed to re-establish acid–base balance.

Renal compensation of respiratory disorders depends primarily upon associated changes in arterial plasma PCO_2 and secondarily upon the resultant alterations in tubular cellular H^+ and activity of the $Na^+–H^+$ antiport: the essential steps are shown in Figure 2.3. Increased arterial plasma PCO_2 also leads to compensatory elevation of plasma HCO_3^- (and vice versa) and, thus, to an increased filtered load of HCO_3^-; under experimental conditions it is possible to demonstrate increased HCO_3^- reabsorption by acutely raising plasma PCO_2. However, renal compensation of respiratory disorders is inevitably slower than the converse. Increased levels of urinary $H_2PO_4^-$ are not normally detectable within six hours of the onset of respiratory acidosis, and take several days to reach maximum level. Thus, the kidneys are better adapted to dealing with chronic than with acute respiratory disorders. The compensatory processes involved are shown in Figure 2.5. Note that, given sufficient time, the kidneys can effect complete compensation (i.e. return pH to 7.4); the lungs are unable completely to compensate for metabolic disturbances.

Not only the onset but also the 'switch-off' of renal compensation is slow, which can lead to over-compensation of the original respiratory imbalance. Thus, post-hypercapnic metabolic alkalosis and post-hypocapnic metabolic acidosis may follow, respectively, respiratory acidosis and alkalosis.

Hypercapnia, in which arterial CO_2 rises above 6 kPa (resulting, for example, from chronic bronchitis, chest damage or the use of respiratory depressant drugs such as barbiturates), will normally lead to a compensatory increase in plasma $[HCO_3^-]$ (as in Figure 2.5). This, however, will raise the delivery of HCO_3^- to the kidney

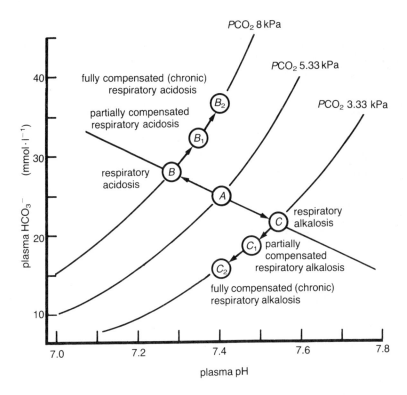

Fig. 2.5 Respiratory acidosis and alkalosis and their renal compensation. Point *A* represents the normal subject (plasma pH 7.4, HCO_3^- 25 mmol·l^{-1}, arterial PCO_2 5.33 kPa). Acidosis moves the point up the true plasma buffer line to *B*, at which plasma pH has fallen, plasma HCO_3^- is slightly elevated, and arterial PCO_2 is markedly elevated. Compensation is partial at B_1 and complete at B_2 (chronic acidosis) due to increased renal H^+ secretion and HCO_3^- reabsorption. Points *C*, C_1 and C_2 show the corresponding response to respiratory alkalosis. Note that the compensation follows the PCO_2 isobars.

in glomerular filtrate; but, provided that the rate of renal H^+ secretion exceeds the rate of HCO_3^- delivery, tubular fluid will become acidified and plasma will remain alkalinised. Conversely, in hypocapnia (arterial $PCO_2 < 4.7$ kPa; occurring, for example, at heights above 3,000 m or during hysterical overbreathing) plasma and filtered HCO_3^- will be compensatorily reduced.

Again, however, net compensation (tubular fluid alkalinisation and sustained plasma acidification) will be achieved so long as the depression of arterial PCO_2 (and, hence, the availability of H^+ for secretion) exceeds the depression of plasma HCO_3^-.

2.6 Potassium and acid–base balance

The distal nephron is the major site of K^+ secretion, as well as of titratable acid. It was at one time believed that the two cations competed for a common secretory mechanism, but this view is no longer tenable as paralled fluctuations in their secretory rates can be demonstrated by appropriate experiments. However, in several circumstances distal K^+ and H^+ secretion do vary reciprocally, K^+ secretion taking place passively down an electrochemical gradient and H^+ secretion occurring by means of the Na^+–H^+ antiport (see 2.3.3.1). In some respects distal cells behave as if they contain a fixed sum, but variable individual amounts, of these cations available for secretion. (This is almost certainly an over-simplification. Intracellular H^+ probably influences the size of the cellular K^+ transport pool via changes in the K^+ permeability of the peritubular membrane, but it remains a useful method of conceptualising the inter-relationship between H^+ and K^+ secretion.) Thus, in extracellular metabolic acidosis, in an individual in normal K^+ balance, an increase in H^+ secretion may lead to inappropriately low levels of distal K^+ secretion and, hence, to hyperkalaemia. Conversely, renal tubular acidosis or the administration of acetazolamide can cause hypokalaemia due to increased K^+ secretion.

In K^+ depletion the lack of the major intracellular cation is probably made good (in all cells, including those of the renal tubule) by accumulation of both Na^+ and H^+. Increased intracellular H^+ does not necessarily involve a significant decrease in pH, since H^+ is buffered by polyanionic macromolecules. In the kidney the extra H^+ will be available for secretion, HCO_3^- reabsorption will thus be increased, and extracellular metabolic alkalosis may result. In K^+ loading there is a decrease in the amount of cellular H^+ available for secretion and HCO_3^- reabsorption is depressed, with the result that cellular fluid remains relatively alkaline in the face of extracellular hyperkalaemic acidosis. These observations make the important point that disturbances in acid–base balance can, under some circumstances, be localised to one or another of the body's fluid compartments.

2.7 Bicarbonate, chloride and the 'anion gap'

The so-called 'anion gap' is the quantitative difference between the plasma concentration of Na^+ and the sum of the concentrations of the major plasma anions, HCO_3^- and Cl^-. It is usually $10–14 \, mmol \cdot l^{-1}$ (or about $4 \, mmol \cdot l^{-1}$ greater if plasma K^+ is taken into account). The gap increases during those metabolic acidotic states which are characterised by production of excess organic or inorganic anions. If these anions are not readily reabsorbable from the glomerular filtrate, homeostatic plasma alkalinisation will be facilitated due to enhanced H^+ secretion in exchange for Na^+.

Alterations in the relative concentrations of HCO_3^- and Cl^- in plasma also have consequences for acid–base balance because of their effects on renal function. Thus, hyperchloraemia is associated with metabolic acidosis because the lack of filtered HCO_3^- depresses H^+ secretion. This is an example of an acidosis which is **not** accompanied by increased 'anion gap'. Conversely, hypochloraemia enhances H^+ secretion and HCO_3^- reabsorption. In both conditions, therefore, the renal response tends to exacerbate the underlying HCO_3^- imbalance by a positive feedback.

2.8 Sodium, diuretics acid–base balance

From consideration of eqn (2.3) and Figure 2.2 it is apparent that acetazolamide should cause metabolic acidosis by depressing HCO_3^- reabsorption. This indeed occurs, although the acidosis tends to be self-limiting, partly due to direct HCO_3^- reabsorption (see 2.3.2.1) and partly due to the fact that when the $[HCO_3^-]$ in plasma and filtrate has fallen to a certain level non-catalytically produced H^+ will be sufficient to maintain a reduced rate of HCO_3^- reabsorption. Because of the relationship between HCO_3^- and Na^+ reabsorption (see 2.3.3), acetazolamide acts as an osmotic diuretic, although its effect in this respect is rather weak.

Unlike acetazolamide, diuretics which impair Na^+ reabsorption in the ascending limb of Henle's loop and in the early distal tubule (the so-called loop diuretics e.g. frusemide, bumetanide and the thiazides) tend to cause alkalosis because they increase delivery of Na^+ to the more distal parts of the nephron and, hence, increase the activity of the Na^+-H^+ antiport (see 2.3.3.1). This alkalosis is accompanied by hypokalaemia, since increased fluid flow in the distal nephron increases the rate at which secreted K^+ is removed from the site of secretion, maintaining a high secretory electro-chemical gradient. There are two further contributory causes to this alkalosis. Diuretics reduce extracellular fluid volume and, hence, raise the concentrations of plasma solutes, including HCO_3^-. They also increase the excretion of Cl^- (as $NaCl$), leading to a potential plasma anion deficit which is filled by HCO_3^-. Alkalosis of this type, like that resulting from prolonged vomiting, can be corrected by administration of Cl^-.

Late distal diuretics such as amiloride and the aldosterone analogue spironolactone may lead to metabolic acidosis (by reducing Na^+-H^+ exchange) and hyperkalaemia (by depressing other Na^+ reabsorptive mechanisms). Similarly, adrenalectomy (which leads to a lack of aldosterone) may cause hyperkalaemic acidosis, while primary hyperaldosteronism leads to hypokalaemic alkalosis. Acid–base (and K^+) imbalance due to diuretic therapy can be minimised of loop and late distal diuretics are administered simultaneously.

2.9 Further reading

R. F. Pitts. *Physiology of the Kidney and Body Fluids*. Year book Medical Publishers. First published in 1963, this book remains essential reading for renal physiologists; the 3rd edition appeared in 1974. The chapters on acid–base balance are of particular interest since the author played a major part in developing our understanding of this aspect of the subject.

C. J. Lote. *Principles of Renal Physiology*. Croom Helm, 1982. A straightforward account of the topic.

J. R. Robinson. *Fundamentals of Acid–Base Regulation*. Black-well Scientific Publications 5th edition, 1975. This specialised text is recommended, although it should be noted that the author's use of the terms 'acidosis' and 'alkalosis' is at variance with that in the present chapter.

Recently published texts with a clinical orientation include:

G. M. Berlyne. *A Course in Clinical Disorders of the Body Fluids and Electrolytes.* Blackwell Scientific Publications, 1980; J. L. Gamble. *Acid–Base Physiology.* John Hopkins University Press, 1982; P. Richards & B. Truniger. *Understanding Water, Electrolyte and Acid–Base Balance.* William Heinemann Medical, 1983.

For a detailed description of specific aspects of renal acid–base regulation the advanced or enquiring student should consult the specialist reviews of which the following is a representative selection:

Dobyan, D. & Bulger, R. W. (1982). Renal carbonic anhydrase. *Amer. J. Physiol.*, **243**, F311–24.

Malnic, G. & Steinmetz, P. R. (1976). Transport processes in urinary acidification. *Kidney int.*, **9**, 172–88.

Maren, T. H. (1974). Chemistry of the renal reabsorption of bicarbonate. *Can. J. Physiol. Pharmacol.*, **52**, 1041–50.

Pitts, R. F. (1973), Production and excretion of ammonia in relation to acid–base regulation. In: *Handbook of Physiology*, Section 8, 455–96 (eds. J. Orloff and R. W. Berliner). American Physiological Society.

Rector, F. C. (1983). Sodium, bicarbonate, and chloride absorption by the proximal tubule. *Amer. J. Physiol.*, **244**, F461–71.

Warnock, D. G. & Rector, F. C. (1979). Proton secretion by the kidney. *Ann. Rev. Physiol.*, **41**, 197 210.

3

Intracellular pH

R. C. Thomas   Department of Physiology, University of Bristol

3.1 Introduction

While the biochemical importance of intracellular pH (pH_i) has been known for a long time, it is only recently that its normal value has been accurately measured and its control mechanisms have begun to be elucidated.

The several different methods now available for measuring pH_i all show it is usually close to the extracellular pH (pH_o) but slightly more acid, typically about 7.2. This means that the free intracellular hydrogen ion concentration $[H^+]$ is less than $100 \, \text{nmol} \cdot l^{-1}$, about a million times less than intracellular $[K^+]$. The H^+ ion is so reactive with proteins and other biochemical compounds that even such a low level of H^+ ions must be tightly controlled to avoid disturbing cell physiology and biochemistry.

In the long term pH_i is kept constant by transport processes that effectively extrude excess acid from the cell but short term changes in pH_i are minimised by buffering. Some pH_i changes may have a role as intracellular signals, but in most cases pH_i is of such wide and fundamental importance that it is kept as constant as possible.

3.2 Methods for measuring pH_i

Ever since its biochemical importance was realised, a wide variety of methods have been used to estimate pH_i in animal (and even plant) cells. The most important methods are outlined in the following sections.

3.2.1 Homogenate pH
This method appeals to biochemists. A tissue sample is rapidly homogenised and its pH measured with a conventional pH

electrode. If the organelles are left intact, and minimal loss of CO_2 occurs, the homogenate pH may be similar to the true cytoplasmic pH.

3.2.2 Weak acid distribution
A labelled weak acid or base is allowed to equilibrate between the inside and outside of the cells. Then its distribution is measured and the pH_i calculated on the assumption that the cell membranes are essentially only permeable to the uncharged molecules. The procedure requires destruction of the tissue and only gives valid answers when the pH_i is stable but has, nevertheless, given much useful information. The most commonly used weak acid is 5, 5-dimethyl-2, 4-oxazolidinedione (DMO).

3.2.3 Intracellular pH indicators
Several natural pigments are pH-sensitive, and they provided the earliest methods for following pH_i changes in plant cells. Conventional pH indicators can be directly injected into large cells, and have been used to investigate pH changes. Perhaps the most ingenious way of getting indicators into cells is first to convert the dye into an inactive ester. This is then readily taken up by the cell and converted back into the active form by naturally occurring intracellular enzymes. Ideally, the active form is trapped intra-cellularly by being impermeant. A currently popular compound for pH_i measurements is dimethylcarboxyfluorescein. Either fluorescence or absorbance can be used to measure pH_i, although calibration can be difficult.

3.2.4 ^{31}P Nuclear magnetic resonance
This powerful but expensive and complex method depends on the intrinsic magnetic properties of the phosphorus (P) atomic nucleus. Its great advantage is that it is non-invasive and measures much more than pH.

The ^{31}P nucleus reacts with a strong magnetic field in such a way that it will absorb and then re-emit radiofrequency radiation with which it resonates. The precise frequency depends on the other elements with which phosphorus is combined. Thus, the frequency for inorganic phosphate is different from that for phosphocreatine. Further, the phosphate frequency depends on the relative amounts

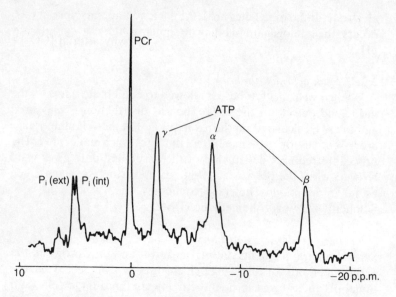

Fig. 3.1 Nuclear magnetic resonance spectrum from a perfused rat heart. Frequency shifts shown in p.p.m. relative to that due to the ^{31}P in phosphocreatine (PCr). The signal was collected over 8 min at 73.8 MHz. The inorganic phosphate (P_i) peak is a double one since the P_i was in two compartments, extracellular and intracellular, which were at two different pHs. (From Grove, T. H., Ackerman, J. J. H., Radda, G. K. & Bore, P. J. (1980) *Proc. Natl. Acad. Sci.* U.S.A., **77**, 299–302)

of the two anions $H_2PO_4^-$ and HPO_4^{2-}, which in turn depends on pH. If all the phosphate is at the same pH the frequency of resonance will give the pH in the phosphate space.

In practice the tissue is placed in a superconducting magnet and zapped every second or so with an intense pulse of radiation with many different frequencies around 100 MHz. After each pulse a signal can be picked up from the phosphorus nuclei. Averaged signals are converted into an n.m.r. spectrum such as that shown in Figure 3.1 by a Fourier transform process. There are peaks for each chemically distinct ^{31}P nucleus, as long as there are significant quantities of each compound.

The advantages of n.m.r. spectroscopy are its non-invasiveness and ability to measure many metabolites as well as pH$_i$ at frequent intervals over long periods of time. However, accurate pH_i measurements require the presence of relatively large amounts of phosphate in the cytoplasm and not elsewhere, and require densely-packed cells to give an adequate signal.

3.2.5 *Microelectrodes sensitive to pH*

It is possible, with experience, to make pH-sensitive microelectrodes suitable for measuring pH_i in large or robust cells. Either pH-sensitive glass, as used in conventional pH electrodes, or a suitable neutral ligand solution can be used as the sensing element. A second reference microelectrode is needed in the same cell to measure the membrane potential, which must be subtracted from the voltage recorded by the pH microelectrode, as shown in Figure 3.2. Rather than two separate electrodes, one double-barrelled microelectrode can be used instead.

The advantages of this method are its simplicity, ease of calibration, and that it gives a continuous recording of the pH at one point inside the cell. The same method can readily be used with other ion-sensitive materials to record other intracellular ion activities. Reliable results, however, depend on the application of rigorous criteria concerning stability of the electrodes, reproductivity of the calibration, completeness of the cell penetration and avoidance of excessive injury.

3.3 **Are H^+ ions passively distributed?**

3.3.1 *The normal pH_i*

A wide variety of preparations have now been investigated with a number of methods for measuring pH_i. It is generally agreed that in most animal cells the normal pH_i is between 7.0 and 7.4, while the external pH is usually slightly higher. Where different methods have been used on the same preparation, good agreement has usually been found. Thus, the pH_i measured with microelectrodes in crab muscle at 20 °C as in Figure 3.2 averaged 7.27, while that measured with the weak acid DMO in barnacle muscle was 7.29. Mammalian muscle at 37 °C tends to have a pH_i closer to 7, but this is partly due to the effect of temperature on the neutral pH of water.

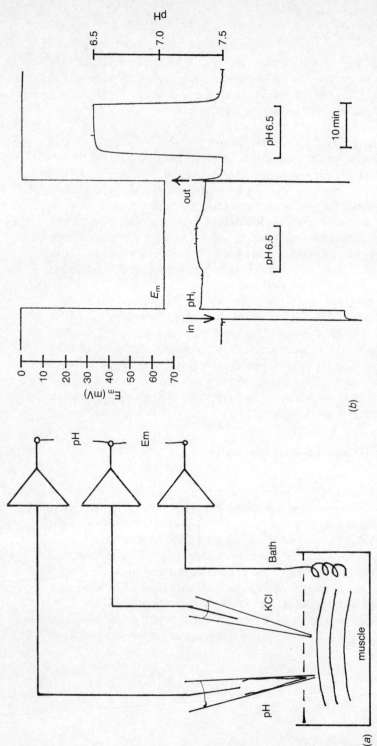

Fig. 3.2 Measuring crab muscle pH_i with microelectrodes. (a) Diagram of the electrode arrangements. (b) Pen recording of the potentials recorded during an experiment. Top line is the voltage from the KCl-filled microelectrode used to measure the membrane potential (E_m), bottom line is the voltage difference between the KCl- and pH- sensitive microelectrodes. The arrow indicates the point on the pH record when the pH electrode was pushed into a fibre. About two minutes later the KCl electrode was pushed into the same fibre, causing the upward jump in the pH record. Except where shown, the fibre was superfused with pH 7.5 saline. At the second arrow both electrodes were

3.3.2 *What is the equilibrium potential for H⁺?*

If pH_o is typically about 7.4, and pH_i about 7.2, the equilibrium potential for H^+ ions (E_H) can be calculated from the Nernst equation

$$E_H = \frac{RT}{nF} \ln \frac{[H]_o}{[H]_i}$$

where R is the gas constant, T the absolute temperature, n is the valency, F the Faraday and $[H]_o$ and $[H]_i$ the external and internal H^+ ion activities. At 20 °C, and converting $[H]$ to 10^{-pH} (since that is how pH was originally defined), converting natural logarithms to logarithms to base 10, and putting in the values of the four constants,

$$E_H = 58 \log(10^{-7.4}/10^{-7.2})$$
$$= 58 \times (-0.2) = -11.6 \, \text{mV}$$

Because of the relationship between H^+, OH^- and HCO_3^-, the equilibrium potentials for all three ions will be the same as long as $[CO_2]$ is the same inside and outside the cell. Figure 3.3 shows the relative values for the various important ions.

Since the equilibrium potential for an ion is the only potential at which passive fluxes in and out of a cell are equal, it is impossible to explain the normal pH_i without invoking some non-passive transport. Somehow energy must be used to expel from the cell the excess passive influx of H^+ ions (or efflux of HCO_3^-) that will result from the difference between the resting potential and E_H. The same transport system will presumably restore pH_i to normal after an acidification.

3.4 External influences on pH_i

3.4.1 *Ions*

Cell membranes are not very permeable to ions, including those associated with pH; namely H^+, OH^- and HCO_3^-. Thus, to some extent the cytoplasm is isolated from the extracellular fluid as far as pH is concerned. (The red blood cell is a special case: its membrane has so many Cl^-/HCO_3^- exchangers that it behaves as

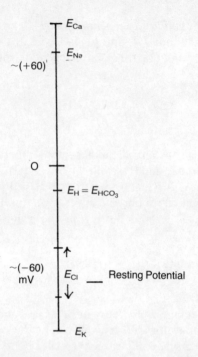

Fig. 3.3 Scale showing relative values of the equilibrium potential (as given by the Nernst equation) for various ions across the membrane of a typical excitable cell. Numerical values on the left are very approximate; the extracellur fluid being taken as zero.

if it were permeable to HCO_3^-. This is important for CO_2 carriage.)

The essential equivalence of these three ions should perhaps be explained. Movement of H^+ ions one way across a membrane is indistinguishable from movement of OH^- ions in the opposite direction, and, since in life CO_2 is always present, HCO_3^- and OH^- ions are also equivalent. This is due to the reaction

$$CO_2 + H_2O \rightleftharpoons H_2CO_3 \rightleftharpoons H^+ + HCO_3^-$$

This reaction is slow in the absence of carbonic anhydrase, but since this enzyme is very widely distributed it is unlikely that the reaction's slowness is ever a problem. Thus, when CO_2 levels are

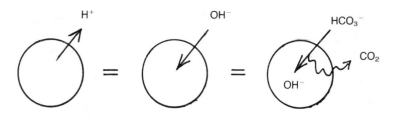

Fig. 3.4 Diagram showing ion movements which would have the same effect on pH_i.

constant, H^+ efflux is equivalent to OH^- or HCO_3^- influx, as shown in Figure 3.4. At normal pH and CO_2 levels, there are about 10^5 times more HCO_3^- ions than OH^- ions, per unit volume.

None of these ions appear to cross cell membranes very rapidly. When pH_o is changed either at constant or zero CO_2 levels, there are only slow and small effects on pH_i, as shown in Figure 3.2. A long exposure to an abnormal pH_o may eventually cause a large pH_i change, but this may be more due to interference with pH_i regulation than to passive ion movements (see also section 3.7.2).

3.4.2 *Weak acids and bases*

Although cell membranes are poorly permeable to ions, they are highly permeable to small uncharged molecules. The uncharged molecules which are important as far as pH_i is concerned are the undissociated molecules of weak acids, such as carbonic, lactic and acetic acid, and also some weak bases. Hydrated CO_2, or carbonic acid, is probably the most important weak acid. There are about five hundred CO_2 molecules in solution for every carbonic acid molecule. The reactions and movements of molecules that occur when a cell is exposed to CO_2, to acetic acid, and to the weak base NH_3 are shown in Figure 3.5.

The production of intracellular H^+ ions by the weak acid (or consumption of H^+ by the base) can cause a large and rapid pH_i change. An example of this is shown in Figure 3.6 from an experiment on a snail neurone. The entry of CO_2 rapidly causes pH_i to decrease by over half a pH unit, and there is an equally rapid recovery when the CO_2 is removed. The extent to which

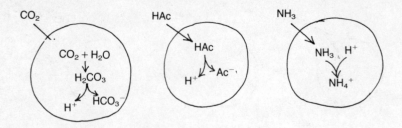

Fig. 3.5 Diagram showing how CO_2 and acetic acid (HAc) cause a decrease in pH_i by producing H^+ ions inside the cell, and how ammonia causes an initial rise in pH_i by consuming H^+ ions. Long exposure to ammonia leads to a pH_i decrease as NH_4^+ ions enter through cation channels and eventually cause an efflux of ammonia.

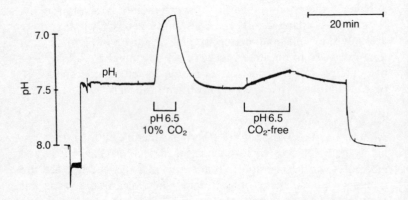

Fig. 3.6 The effect of 10 per cent CO_2 on snail neurone pH_i recorded with a pH-sensitive microelectrode. The external pH was 8 except where indicated. The CO_2 was applied at pH 6.5 so a CO_2-free Ringer solution of the same pH was applied as a control. (From Thomas, R. C. (1974) *J. Physiol.*, **238**, 159–80.)

changes in extracellular levels of weak acids and bases occur physiologically are largely unknown, but they are potentially much more important than pH_o in influencing pH_i. Similarly, metabolically produced weak acids such as lactic acid may have large effects on pH_i, both in the cell producing the acid and on neighbouring cells.

3.4.3 *Membrane potential*

At rest the cell membrane is relatively impermeable to H^+ and other ions, and pH_i is only slowly changed by changing pH_o. Changing the membrane potential might also be expected to have little effect on pH_i, and this has been shown for increases in membrane potential (Em) for a number of preparations. Thus, increasing E_m from -50 mV to -100 mV had no effect on snail neurone pH_i.

Rather surprisingly, however, large decreases of Em, especially to values where the cytoplasm is positive to the exterior, appear to increase greatly the membrane's permeability to H^+ ions, so much so that if the potential is held positive for many seconds pH_i becomes sensitive to E_m. The physiological significance of this apparent appearance of proton permeable channels is unknown (see Thomas & Meech, 1982).

3.5 **Intracellular buffering**

In the short term (seconds rather than minutes) pH_i changes are minimised by intracellular buffering. This term includes several different mechanisms that rapidly consume or release H^+ when acid or alkali are added to the cytoplasm. The main mechanisms are (*a*) chemical buffering, in which the salts of weak acids and bases combine with H^+ ions to make undissociated compounds, (*b*) biochemical conversion of metabolic acids to non-acid compounds and (*c*) movement of acid or alkali between the cytoplasm and the interior of various organelles. Little is known about the relative importance of the last two mechanisms, but chemical buffering is probably the most important of the three.

It must be stressed that buffering **reduces** pH_i changes, but cannot prevent them. Biochemical reactions or ion transport may later return the pH_i to its previous level, but such pH_i recovery is not part of buffering.

3.5.1 *The importance of pK*

As described in Chapter 1, strong acids and bases ionise completely in aqueous solution; weak acids and bases do not. Thus, a solution of a weak acid (HA), such as lactic acid, contains two components more than pure water: HA and A^-. The dissociation of HA can be written:

$$HA \rightleftharpoons H^+ + A^-$$

From the law of mass action the equilibrium constant K is given by

$$K = \frac{[H^+] \times [A^-]}{[HA]}$$

Rearranging this, taking the logarithm of both sides and putting pK equal to the negative log of K gives the important Henderson–Hasselbalch equation:

$$pH = pK + \log\frac{[A^-]}{[HA]}$$

From this it is clear that the pK is the pH at which the weak acid HA is half ionised. It is at this pH that a weak acid is at its most effective as a buffer, as first shown by Koppel and Spiro in 1914.

Buffering power (β) is defined as the amount of strong base required to change the pH of one litre of solution by one pH unit. At its pK a $1 \, mol \cdot l^{-1}$ solution of a monovalent weak acid has a buffering power of $0.58 \, mol \cdot pH^{-1} \cdot l^{-1}$. Putting this another way, the maximum molar buffer value of a single ionisable group is 0.58 per pH unit.

3.5.2 *Measuring intracellular buffering power*

Two different methods have been used to measure intracellular buffering power. In one, strong acid is added directly to the cell interior by microinjection and the pH_i change measured, but this is only applicable to large cells. In the other, more widely applicable, method the pH_i is recorded while the cell is exposed to a well-buffered solution containing CO_2, NH_3 or another weak acid or base. When the pH_i stops changing it is assumed that the internal and external levels of the permeant species are equal.

Perhaps this can best be explained by means of an example as shown in Figure 3.7, in which a cell is exposed to $10 \, mmol \cdot l^{-1}$ propionate. Having recorded the pH_i changes, the next step is to calculate the undissociated propionic acid (H Prop) level outside the cell. The pH_o is 7.5, and the pK for propionic acid is 4.87.

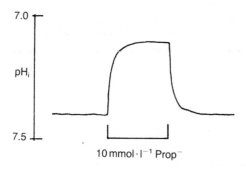

Fig. 3.7 Expected pH_i record from model experiment to measure intracellular buffering power. External pH 7.5. Propionate applied for about 5 min. No pH_i regulation.

Putting these values into the Henderson–Hasselbalch equation gives

$$7.5 - 4.87 = \log \frac{0.01}{[\mathrm{H\,Prop}]}$$

Thus

$$[\mathrm{H\,Prop}] = 0.01/(\text{antilog}\,2.63)$$
$$= 2.3 \times 10^{-5}$$

i.e. the undissociated propionic acid concentration is $23\,\mu\mathrm{mol}\cdot\mathrm{l}^{-1}$.

In the example the steady pH_i in the presence of propionate is 7.1. Presumably the internal $[\mathrm{H\,Prop}]$ is now also $23\,\mu\mathrm{mol}\cdot\mathrm{l}^{-1}$. Again using the Henderson–Hasselbalch equation, this gives an intracellular propionate level of $3.9\,\mathrm{mmol}\cdot\mathrm{l}^{-1}$. Since this is all presumed to have entered the cell as H Prop, the propionate must have been accompanied by $3.9\,\mathrm{mmol}\cdot\mathrm{l}^{-1}$ of H^+, which caused a pH_i decrease of 0.3 unit. Thus, β_i was $3.9/0.3 = 13\,\mathrm{mmol}\cdot\mathrm{pH}^{-1}\cdot\mathrm{l}^{-1}$. Values obtained experimentally range from 9 for squid axons to over 100 for striated muscle, the high values for muscle presumably reflecting its high protein content. Many early measurements of β_i were distorted by a failure to allow for pH_i regulation.

As well as minimising pH_i changes, intracellular buffering may be important in determining the intracellular mobility of H^+ ions. Looking at it backwards, β is a measure of H^+ availability, and may be an important factor in keeping pH_i uniform throughout the cytoplasm.

3.5.3 *Buffering power when external CO_2 is fixed*
The pK for the dissociation of carbonic acid is about 6.1, too far from the normal pH_i for bicarbonate to be an important buffer unless the CO_2 level is fixed. If the external $[CO_2]$ is kept constant, as it generally would be *in vivo*, the cell membrane is so permeable to CO_2 that at least in small cells internal $[CO_2]$ would be kept constant too.

In this situation, first recognised by Van Slyke in the 1920s, internal bicarbonate becomes a very powerful buffer: its buffering power at any pH is four times that of other buffers at their pK, on a mole for mole basis. An example of this effect of external CO_2 is shown in Figure 3.8. In this experiment β_i was determined by NH_4Cl injection, which is equivalent to HCl injection since the NH_4^+ dissociates to H^+ and NH_3, and the latter readily leaves the cell. In the absence of CO_2, β_i was about $12 \, \text{mmol} \cdot pH^{-1} \cdot l^{-1}$, but in the presence of CO_2 the β_i was 48: a rather spectacular increase.

Permeant compounds other than CO_2 which are kept constant extracellularly by the circulation could also contribute to intracellular buffering, although at present no evidence is available for any such contribution. Perhaps buffering is too boring to have been studied by physiologists as much as it deserves.

3.6 **Intracellular pH regulation**

While buffering minimises pH_i changes, any restoration of pH_i after an acidification (such as that caused by NH_4Cl injection or CO_2 application, shown in Figure 3.8) requires some sort of active transport process. Until 1975 virtually nothing was known about the mechanism of pH_i regulation, and indeed there was then still some argument about whether or not a special transport system was needed.

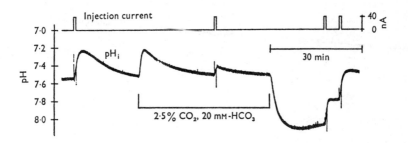

Fig. 3.8 Experiment on snail neurone pH_i to show the effect of CO_2 on the intracellular buffering power, which was measured by brief injections of NH_4Cl as shown on the upper line. The first, third and fourth injections were made with the cell bathed with CO_2-free Ringer solution, pH 7.5, and the second made with the cell in Ringer solution of the same pH equilibrated with 2.5 per cent CO_2. The bottom line shows the pH_i recorded with a pH-sensitive microelectrode. (From Thomas, R. C. (1974) *J. Physiol.*, **241**, 103P–104P.)

3.6.1 *Various ionic mechanisms*

Most studies of the mechanism of pH_i regulation have concentrated on pH_i recovery from acidification, since passive ion fluxes would tend to acidify pH_i. Experimentally the acidification has been achieved either by acid injection, by loading the cell with NH_4^+ ions, or by increasing CO_2.

So far the ionic mechanism of the acid extrusion which occurs as pH_i recovers from acidification has only been elucidated in a small number of preparations. Nevertheless, there appear to be at least three different ionic mechanisms for acid extrusion, as shown in Figure 3.9. These are Cl^-/HCO_3^- exchange, Na^+/H^+ exchange, and Na^+-dependent Cl^-/HCO_3^- exchange. The last may involve H^+ movement too, as shown in Figure 3.9. All three mechanisms are electrically neutral.

3.6.2 *Snail neurones, squid axon and barnacle muscle*

Because of their large size these preparations were the first to be investigated in detail with pH-sensitive microelectrodes. It was discovered in 1976 that pH_i recovery in squid axons and snail neurones was faster in the presence of bicarbonate, as shown in Figure 3.10a. It was also found that anion exchange inhibitors,

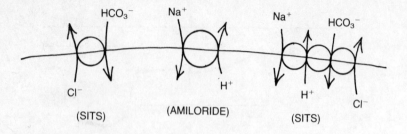

Fig. 3.9 Ionic mechanisms for pH_i regulation. (Blocking agents shown in parentheses.)

such as SITS, that blocked Cl^-/HCO_3^- exchange in red blood cells, blocked pH_i recovery in snail neurones and squid axons. The removal of internal Cl^- also blocked pH_i recovery, suggesting that the mechanism might be a simple Cl^-/HCO_3^- exchanger. This suggestion turned out to be too good to be true because the removal of external Na^+ also blocked pH_i recovery, as shown in Figure 3.10. Sodium entry was found to be increased during pH_i recovery. In all three preparations it is now thought that pH_i regulation is either by a Na^+–dependent Cl^-/HCO_3^- exchanger or, as originally proposed, a four-ion carrier transporting Cl^- and H^+ ions out of the cell in exchange for HCO_3^- and Na^+ ions carried in. The Na^+ gradient apparently supplies the energy, although in squid axons ATP is required.

3.6.3 *Vertebrate cells*
Probably the first mammalian preparation in which the mechanism of pH_i regulation was established was mouse skeletal muscle. Aickin recorded pH_i with pH glass microelectrodes and found that recovery from acidification was greatly slowed by removal of external Na^+ or by application of the diuretic amiloride. Internal $[Na^+]$ changed in a way consistent with its entry in exchange for H^+. Anion exchange inhibitors or CO_2 removal caused some slowing of pH_i recovery, additive to the effects of Na^+ removal. It appeared that the major mechanism for pH_i recovery was Na^+/H^+ exchange, with a separate involvement (about 20 per cent) of Cl^-/HCO_3^- exchange.

Many investigations of other vertebrate preparations have been

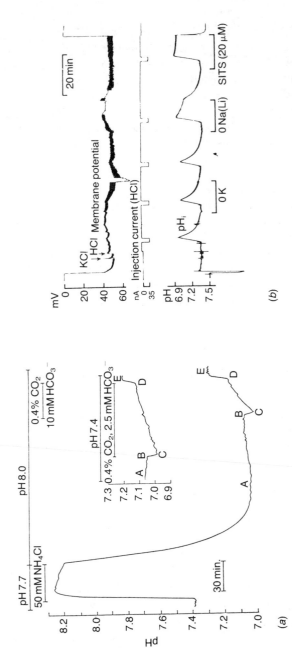

Fig. 3.10 Investigations of pH$_i$ regulation. (a) Upside-down experiment on squid giant axon showing that pH$_i$ recovery after ammonium-induced acidification is accelerated by HCO$_3^-$. Section AB of the pH$_i$ record shows recovery without, and section CD with, bicarbonate. Inset from similar experiment at lower external pH. (From Boron, W. F. & De Weer, P. (1976) *Nature*, **259**, 240–41, reproduced with permission.) (b) Experiment on snail neurone showing pH$_i$ recovery after HCl injection is inhibited by replacing external Na with Li, and blocked by SITS. (From Thomas, R. C. (1976) *J. Physiol.*, **263**, 212–13P.)

done in the absence of HCO_3^-, so the extent of Cl^-/HCO_3^- involvement in pH_i recovery is obscure. It may be important in pH_i recovery from alkalinisation. In all cases, however, it is clear that amiloride-sensitive Na^+/H^+ exchange plays a major role. This has been shown with microelectrodes in sheep heart Purkinje fibres, salamander kidney and lamprey neurones and with fluorescent indicators in mammal fibroblasts and lymphocytes, and rabbit kidney tubules. An experiment from the last is shown in Figure 3.11.

3.6.4 *Crayfish and leech neurones*
Crayfish neurone pH_i regulation was investigated by Moody using pH-sensitive glass microelectrodes. He found that pH_i recovery was totally inhibited by removing external Na^+, but only partially by removing HCO_3^-, or by applying SITS. He concluded that there were two independent mechanisms, one being Na^+/H^+ exchange as in vertebrates, the other a Na^+-dependent Cl^-/HCO_3^- exchange as in snail neurones. Recent work suggests that a similar dual mechanism is responsible for pH_i regulation by leech neurones.

3.7 **Intracellular pH changes in ischaemia, acidosis and alkalosis**

The pathophysiology of pH_i has been relatively little investigated so far, although the wider use of n.m.r. methods should make pH_i measurements *in vivo* more attainable. The effects of anoxia or ischaemia, in which a tissue is deprived of oxygen by blocking its blood supply, have already been studied to some extent.

3.7.1 *Ischaemia*
In the heart, when the blood flow through the coronary arteries is reduced there is a rapid reduction in ventricular contractility. With total stoppage of blood flow recent n.m.r. measurements on rat heart have shown that pH_i falls from 7.05 to 6.2 in 13 min, but the correlation between pH_i decrease and loss of contractility is not close. If blood flow is reduced by only half, pH_i remains virtually normal, although there is a 40 per cent reduction in ventricular pressure.

With skeletal muscle, n.m.r. studies have suggested that ischaemia causes an initial increase in pH_i, presumably as

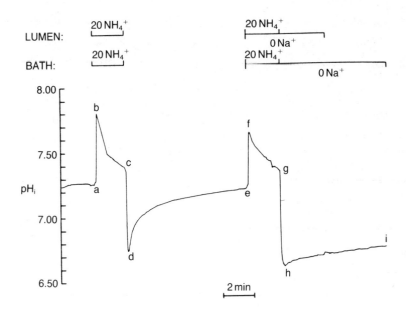

Fig. 3.11 Dye spectrophotometric study of pH$_i$ regulation in rabbit kidney tubule. Absorbance of 4', 5'-dimethyl-5 (and -6) -carboxy-fluorescein used to follow pH$_i$ in isolated perfused cortical collecting tubule. Note upside down pH scale. Recovery from ammonium-induced acidification (d–e) is blocked by removal of Na$^+$ (h–i). (From Chaillet, J. R., Lopes, A. G. & Boron, W. F. (1985) *J. Gen. Physiol.*, in press. Reproduced by copyright permission of the Rockefeller University Press.)

phosphocreatine is broken down. Long periods of ischaemia cause pH$_i$ (measured with microelectrodes) to fall, due to the hydrolysis of ATP and the production of lactic acid. For example, in rabbit muscle pH$_i$ fell from 7.0 to 6.6 during 4 h of ischaemia. During the same period external pH$_i$ fell from 7.3 to 6.4 (Hagberg, 1985).

Nuclear magnetic resonance studies on human kidneys show that pH$_i$ decreases during cold ischaemia to about 6.5 in 24 h. Hypertonic citrate flushed through the kidneys before cold storage prevented much of this decrease in pH$_i$.

3.7.2 *Acidosis and alkalosis*
Understanding metabolic and respiratory acidosis and alkalosis is a major topic for all students of acid–base physiology and it may,

therefore, seem surprising that very little is known about the corresponding pH_i changes. Recent work on mammalian muscle *in vitro*, however, allows some conclusions to be drawn about the probable pH_i effects of changing blood pH.

Figure 3.12 shows two recent experiments on smooth muscle pH_i which contrast the effects of model 'metabolic' (i.e. constant CO_2) alkalosis and acidosis (Figure 3.12a) with those of CO_2 changes (Figure 3.12b). As seen in other preparations also, if CO_2 is kept constant pH_i changes quite slowly by about one third the amount that pH_o is changed. This presumably reflects an effect on pH_i regulation, which depends on other factors as well as the pH difference across the cell membrane.

If CO_2 alone is changed, pH_o being kept constant, there are in all preparations fast transient pH_i changes usually followed by a return to the previous pH_i. In smooth muscle, when CO_2 is removed, the initial pH_i increase is, unusually, followed by a slow fall to a new steady state value. Generally pH_i is independent of the CO_2 level, and even in smooth muscle steady state pH_i was the same in 3 per cent, 5 per cent and 7 per cent CO_2 when pH_o was kept at 7.35.

In respiratory acidosis or alkalosis the speed of the CO_2-induced pH_i change will be combined with the steady state pH_i change seen in metabolic disturbances. Thus, whatever the cause of the pH_o change, the steady-state pH_i change will probably be similar, and about one third of the pH_o change. Given the high intracellular buffering power and the large intracellular volume, the cytoplasm *in vivo* is capable of absorbing a major fraction of any acid or alkali added to the whole body.

3.8 The H^+ ion as an intracellular messenger

There is a widespread belief among researchers that if they can measure something it must be very important. Nevertheless, pH_i is perhaps so biochemically fundamental that it is unlikely to be changed physiologically as some sort of intracellular signal. In fact, a number of examples of the effects of pH_i on membrane channels and intracellular processes have been discovered which could be important physiologically, rather than pathologically. (Any pH_i change of more than about half a unit is likely to occur *in vivo* rather rarely.)

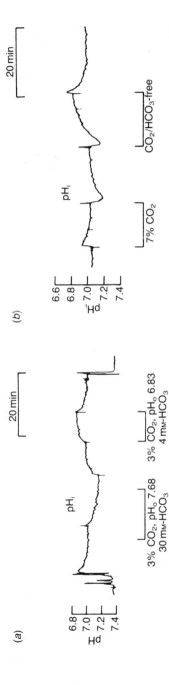

Fig. 3.12 The effect of changing pH_o on pH_i in guinea-pig vas deferens smooth muscle; pH_i measured with double-barrelled pH-sensitive microelectrodes. (a) The effect of changing pH_o without changing CO_2. The pH_o was 7.35 except where indicated, CO_2 was 3 per cent throughout. (b) Changing CO_2 while keeping pH_o constant at 7.35. CO_2 was 3 per cent except where indicated. (From Aickin, C. C. (1984) *J. Physiol.*, **349**, 571–85.)

3.8.1 *Activation of quiescent cells by fertilization, growth factors etc.*

Egg fertilization activates a great variety of metabolic processes, and for some time it was suspected that pH_i changes might be a trigger. In 1976 Johnson, Epel and Paul showed that fertilization of sea urchin eggs was followed by an apparent pH_i increase that could be blocked by amiloride. They suggested that the pH_i increase was due to Na^+/H^+ exchange and played a key role in activating the egg. This suggestion has since received much support from further experiments. Many of the events normally following fertilization can be initiated in the absence of fertilization by an imposed pH_i increase.

Similarly, sperm activation in a variety of species and recovery from dormancy of encysted brine shrimps also appear to involve pH_i increases. The reverse process, the transition from normal development of brine shrimp cysts to anaerobic dormancy was shown in 1982 by Busa and co-workers using ^{31}P-n.m.r. to involve an intracellular acidification of more than 1 pH unit. (They claim a record for any cell pH_i changes under 'biologically meaningful' conditions.) There is some evidence that pH_i changes during the cell cycle may be important in influencing the rate of DNA replication, but it is uncertain as yet that pH_i plays any key role in cell cycle control.

A number of growth factors and tumour-promoting mitogens such as phorbol esters will stimulate cell division in quiescent cell cultures. Recent work by Moolenaar and Grinstein and their respective co-workers suggests that these agents all cause a significant pH_i increase which may be the key stimulus to cell activation. The way the agents work seems to be by binding to a receptor which initiates an inositol phosphate cascade reaction which somehow activates protein kinase C. In turn this aroused enzyme somehow stimulates the amiloride-sensitive Na^+/H^+ exchanger to re-set the normal pH_i to a higher value. It is not yet known whether the pH_i increase that results is really necessary to trigger cell growth. It may simply be that a more active Na^+/H^+ exchanger is required to maintain pH_i during the increased metabolism which follows activation.

The hormone insulin is an important metabolic regulator, and may stimulate glycolysis by means of its effect on pH_i. Extensive studies by Moore show that insulin applied to frog skeletal muscle raises pH_i by 0.1–0.2 units, probably by stimulating Na^+/H^+ exchange. The subsequent stimulation of glycolysis may be mediated by the enzyme phosphofructokinase which is unusually sensitive to pH.

3.8.2 *Barnacle photoreceptor adaptation*
Microelectrode investigations of the response to light by barnacle photoreceptors have revealed that light decreases pH_i, as shown in Figure 3.13*a*. When the pH_i was changed by exposure to CO_2, the response to brief light flashes changed roughly in parallel with the pH_i, as shown in Figure 3.13*b*. Thus, a decrease in pH_i reduced the response to light. Since light itself reduces pH_i, the pH_i decrease could be the mechanism which causes the reduction in sensitivity which occurs with prolonged illumination.

3.8.3 *Membrane channels closed by a fall in pH_i*
A number of ion channels in the cell membrane are sensitive to pH_i changes which might be in the physiological range, and which might be important in the functioning of the cell.

Many, if not most, cells are electrically coupled to their neighbours by channels in their plasma membranes. Loewenstein and his colleagues showed in the 1960s that coupling between insect salivary gland and other cells could be blocked by raising intracellular Ca^{2+}. Later Turin and Warner showed that embryo cells could be uncoupled by exposing them to high levels of CO_2, which caused a decrease in pH_i. The question arose as to whether Ca^{2+} too might work by reducing pH_i, since Ca^{2+} injection into snail neurones had been shown to reduce pH_i. Experiments on cells pairs from fish embryos have shown that the intercellular channels are much more sensitive to H^+ than Ca^{2+} ions. Whether this effect of pH is the mechanism by which cells uncouple physiologically is unknown.

Another channel closed by acidification is a K^+ channel in crayfish muscle fibres which normally prevents action potentials by swamping any depolarising current. Moody has shown that acidification allows the slow muscle fibres to generate all-or-none Ca^{2+} action potentials. Whether this event occurs physiologically is unknown, although the pH_i decrease of about 0.6 which is

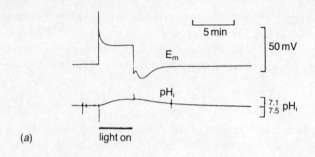

(a)

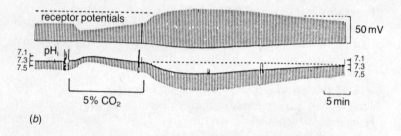

(b)

Fig. 3.13 Barnacle photoreceptor response to light and pH_i measured with a pH-sensitive microelectrode. (*a*) Photoreceptor membrane potential (E_m) and pH_i response to a long period of bright light. The pH_i decreases by 0.16 units. (*b*) The effect of CO_2 on the response to repeated 800 ms light flashes and on the pH_i. (From Brown, H. M. & Meech, R. W. (1979) *J. Physiol.*, **297**, 73–93.)

required seems rather large to occur naturally. Is it an advantage to an anoxic crayfish that its slow muscle fibre should become fast?

If insulin exerts its effect via pH_i, it also seems that pH_i changes may be involved in insulin release. High glucose levels may reduce the pH_i of pancreatic islet cells by stimulating glycolysis. Intracellular acidification of these cells has been shown recently to reduce the open time of K^+ channels, and maybe this changes electrical activity in such a way as to increase insulin release.

3.9 Further reading

Reviews and two books with wide coverage of various topics:
Boron, W. F. & Aronsen, P. S. (1986). Eds. 'Na–H exchange,

intracellular pH, and cell function'. *Current topics in membranes and transport.* Academic Press, New York.

Boron, W. F. (1983). Transport of H^+ and of ionic weak acids and bases. *J. Membrane Biol.* **72**, 1–16.

Busa, W. B. & Nuccitelli, R. (1984). Metabolic regulation via intracellular pH. *Amer. J. Physiol.* **246**, R409–38.

Moody, W. (1984). Effects of intracellular H^+ on the electrical properties of excitable cells. *Ann. Rev. Neurosci.* **7**, 257–78.

Nuccitelli, R. & Deamer, D. W. (1982). Eds. *Intracellular pH: its measurement, regulation and utilization in cellular functions.* Alan R. Liss, New York.

Roos, A. & Boron, W. F. (1981). Intracellular pH. *Physiol. Revs.* **61**, 296–434.

Thomas, R. C. (1984). Experimental displacement of intracellular pH and the mechanism of its subsequent recovery. *J. Physiol.* **354**, 3P–22P.

Other references:

Aickin, C. C. & Thomas, R. C. (1977). An investigation of the ionic mechanism of intracellular pH regulation in mouse soleus muscle fibres. *J. Physiol.* **273**, 295–316.

Busa, W. B., Crowe, J. H. & Matson, G. B. (1982). Intracellular pH and the metabolic status of dormant and developing *Artemia* embryos. *Arch. Biochem. Biophys.* **216**, 711–18.

Chester, M. & Nicholson, C. (1985). Regulation of intracellular pH in vertebrate central neurons. *Brain Research* **325**, 313–16.

Grinstein, S., Rothstein, A. & Cohen, S. (1985). Mechanism of osmotic activation of Na^+/H^+ exchange in rat thymic lymphocytes. *J. Gen. Physiol.* **85**, 765–87.

Hagberg, H. (1985). Intracellular pH during ischemia in skeletal muscle: relationship to membrane potential, extracellular pH, tissue lactic acid and ATP. *Pflügers Archiv.* in press.

Koppel, M. & Sprio, K. (1914). Über die Wirkung von Moderatoren (Puffern) bei der Verschiebung des Säure-Basengleichgewichtes in biologischen Flüssigkeiten. *Biochem. Z.* **65**, 409–34.

Moolenaar, W. H., Tsien, R. Y., Van der Saag, P. T. & De Laat, S. W. (1983). Na^+/H^+ exchange and cytoplasmic pH in the action of growth factors in human fibroblasts. *Nature* **304**, 645–8.

Thomas, R. C. & Meech, R. W. (1982). Hydrogen ion currents and intracellular pH in depolarised voltage-clamped snail neurons. *Nature* **299**, 826–8.

Van Slyke, D. D. (1922). On the measurement of buffer values and on the relationship of buffer value to the dissociation constant of the buffer and the concentration and the reaction of the buffer solution. *J. Biol. Chem.* **52**, 525–70.

Acid–base control in the whole body

R. Hainsworth   Department of Cardiovascular Studies,
University of Leeds

4.1 Importance of acid–base control

Metabolism in the body continuously forms acid (see section
1.1.1). Quantitatively, by far the most important acid to be formed
in this way is carbonic acid; about 10–20 mol of CO_2 must be
removed by the lung each day. Non-volatile acids are formed by
metabolism of foods which results in an excess of sulphuric,
phosphoric or organic acids. The rate of production of these acids
largely depends on the type and quantity of the dietary intake; a
typical value on a western diet is about $60\,\text{mmol}\cdot\text{day}^{-1}$. Non-
volatile acids are partly buffered by the various buffer systems in
the body, in particular haemoglobin ($H^+ + Hb^- \rightleftharpoons HHb$), but they
are mainly neutralised by titration of the bicarbonate buffer:

$$H^+ + HCO_3^- \rightleftharpoons H_2CO_3 \rightleftharpoons H_2O + CO_2$$

Thus, strong acids reduce the amount of bicarbonate buffer and
this can be regenerated only by the kidney. The mechanisms by
which this is achieved are described in Chapter 2. Therefore, the
effect on the body's pH of the addition or removal of acid depends
in the short term on the concentrations of buffers present in the
body and the response by the lung and, in the longer term, on the
response by the kidney.

   In humans, the normal values of pH lie between 7.36 and 7.44;
that is, H^+ concentrations of $44–36\,\text{nmol}\cdot\text{l}^{-1}$. Similar values have
been reported in many other species including dogs, cats, rats,
rabbits and sheep. However, in some species including cats and
rabbits, although similar values of pH are reported, the values of
PCO_2 are lower. The range of pH which is compatible with life for

more than a short period of time is about 7.0–7.7. In terms of pH units this range seems quite narrow, but in terms of $[H^+]$ it actually extends from 100 to 20 $nmol \cdot l^{-1}$.

4.2 Some definitions used in acid–base balance

Acidaemia. The concentration of hydrogen ions in the arterial blood is abnormally high, i.e. pH is abnormally low (<7.36).

Alkalaemia. There is an abnormally low concentration of hydrogen ions in arterial blood, i.e. pH is high (>7.44).

Respiratory acidaemia and alkalaemia. The acidaemia or alkalaemia is the result of a change in $[H^+]$ due to an excessively high $[CO_2]$ (hypercapnia) or a low $[CO_2]$ (hypocapnia).

Non-respiratory (or metabolic) acidaemia and alkalaemia. The acidaemia or alkalaemia is the result of a change in $[H^+]$ due to mechanisms other than changes in $[CO_2]$. They are due to increased or decreased amounts of strong acid or excessive loss or gain of base.

Base excess and base deficit. These are measures of the non-respiratory component of an acid–base disorder. Base excess is the amount of strong acid required to titrate one litre of blood to a pH of 7.4 with PCO_2 of 5.3 kPa at body temperature. Base deficit is the amount of strong base required to titrate one litre of blood to a pH of 7.4 with PCO_2 of 5.3 kPa.

Non-respiratory pH. This is another quantitative measure of the severity of a non-respiratory acidaemia or alkalaemia. For method of determination see page 85.

4.3 Physiological consequences of acid–base disturbances

Acid–base disturbances occur in several diseases of metabolism and in disorders of the kidney, the lung and the heart. Changes in acid–base status are also likely to occur in anaesthetised animal preparations. Most commonly used general anaesthetics cause some depression of respiration and, thus, an increase in PCO_2 and decrease in pH. Prolonged experimental procedures tend to result in a progressive non-respiratory acidaemia. The degree of acidaemia is related to the degree of surgical trauma and is probably due to the underperfusion of some tissues.

The clinical manifestations of acidaemia or alkalaemia are likely to be confused by the effects of the underlying clinical condition (see also Chapter 5). Changes in pH and PCO_2 in the blood, both below and above normal values, have important effects on metabolic processes and on the function of the various systems of the body.

Clinically, acidaemic patients may show an increase in the rate and, particularly, the depth of breathing, often with a hissing noise (Kussmaul's breathing), due to stimulation of the respiratory control centres. Patients may complain of fatigue, headaches and weakness. Severe acidaemia leads to impaired consciousness, delirium, coma and death. In alkalaemia there may be signs of an increased irritability of the central and peripheral nervous systems with paraesthesia and possibly tetany. Frequently, changes in $[H^+]$ are accompanied by directionally similar changes in $[K^+]$ and many of the symptoms of acidaemia or alkalaemia may be attributable, at least in part, to the concomitant changes in potassium. Indeed, one of the dangers of severe acidaemia is the development of cardiac arrhythmias, in particular intraventricular conduction defects, block and ventricular fibrillation, which are probably mainly due to the raised potassium level.

The effects of acid–base disorders on the cardiovascular system are complex. There are direct actions on the heart and blood vessels, reflex effects mediated by peripheral chemoreceptors and effects brought about by an action directly on the central nervous system. Carbon dioxide and hydrogen ions exert a direct vasodilatory action on vascular smooth muscle. Their importance varies in different regions. For example, the level of CO_2 has been shown to be particularly important in the control of the cerebral circulation (Lassen, 1974). Severe hypercapnia and acidaemia depress the strength of contraction of the heart. The responses of the cardiovascular system to stimulation of the autonomic nerves are influenced by the acid–base status. Acidaemia reduces or abolishes the responses of the heart to stimulation of sympathetic nerves and enhances the bradycardia due to vagal stimulation. This may influence reflex responses. For example, Harry, Kappagoda, Linden & Snow (1971) stimulated left atrial receptors in the dog, which results in a reflex tachycardia mediated solely by efferent sympathetic nerves, and found that the response was reduced in the presence of respiratory or non-respiratory acidaemia.

An increase in $[H^+]$, with or without hypercapnia, stimulates peripheral chemoreceptors and increases their sensitivity to hypoxia. The reflex effects are an increase in the rate and depth of breathing. If the ventilatory response is prevented, stimulation of carotid chemoreceptors also results in bradycardia and a negative inotropic response of the heart, and constriction of resistance and capacitance vessels. The level of CO_2 and pH of the blood perfusing the cephalic circulation also has a major effect on efferent sympathetic nervous activity. Cephalic hypercapnia and acidaemia result in an increase in the chronotropic and inotropic state of the heart and in constriction of resistance and capacitance vessels. The reflex responses of the heart and blood vessels to stimulation of baroreceptors and chemoreceptors also are increased (e.g. Hainsworth, McGregor, Rankin & Soladoye, 1984). It is important, therefore, when making physiological studies of reflex responses in a human or animal subject, to pay particular attention to the acid–base state.

4.4 Buffering in the blood and extracellular fluid

Many of the concepts of buffering in the body were deduced from the behaviour of samples of blood equilibrated with various levels of CO_2 in a test tube. However, it is now apparent that, even in the short term, the whole body behaves differently from blood in a test tube and, in the longer term, several other compensatory systems and buffers become important.

The buffering of carbonic acid by blood is better than that by the whole body (Figure 4.1). This is because the concentrations of haemoglobin and plasma proteins are three times as great in the blood compared with the blood plus the extracellular fluid. The reaction of CO_2 with H_2O to form carbonic acid takes place mainly in the red cells due to the presence there of carbonic anhydrase (see section 1.5.1) which greatly increases the speed of the reaction. The dissociation of H_2CO_3 into H^+ and HCO_3^- also takes place mainly in the red cells where H^+ ions are buffered by

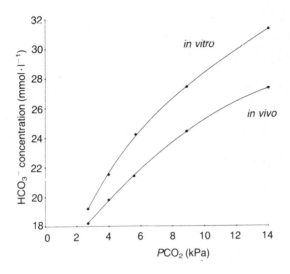

Fig. 4.1 Buffer curves of whole blood (*in vitro*) and whole body (*in vivo*). Note that in the *in vitro* curve the concentrations of HCO_3^- at each value of PCO_2 were greater. This is due to the greater concentration of buffers, in particular haemoglobin, which is able to buffer the H^+ ions and result in a greater production of HCO_3^-. The difference is greatest at high values of PCO_2. (Drawn from data of Levesque, 1975.)

haemoglobin. The concentration of haemoglobin determines the state of the equilibrium. Higher concentrations of haemoglobin displace these reactions to the right; i.e. there would be more HCO_3^- formed but a lower concentration of H^+ ions. Because CO_2 and HCO_3^- become distributed throughout the extracellular fluid, it is possible to consider haemoglobin, which of course is present only in the blood compartment, as if it were present in a lower concentration in the whole extracellular fluid. Therefore, in the extracellular fluid a given change in the level of CO_2 will result in larger changes in pH and smaller changes in HCO_3^- than in blood equilibrated *in vitro*.

Acid–base balance is frequently assessed by the use of nomograms. A commonly used nomogram was described by Siggaard-Andersen in 1962 (Figure 4.2). To use this, values of PCO_2 and pH in arterial blood are determined and a line is drawn between

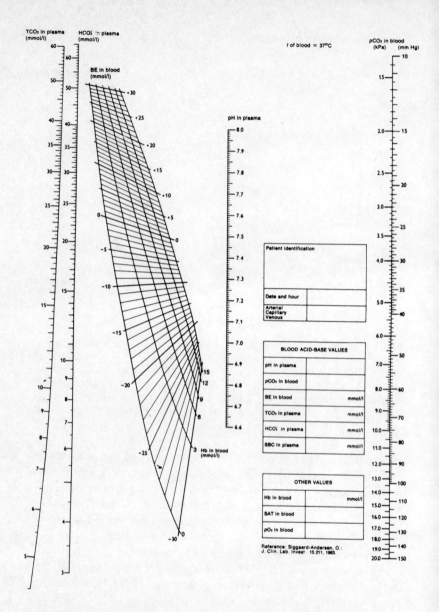

Fig. 4.2 Siggaard-Andersen acid–base nomogram. To use this nomogram align the values of PCO_2 and pH and read the value of base excess (or base deficit) from the line intersecting the appropriate value of the haemoglobin concentration. Note that haemoglobin concentration is given in $mmol \cdot l^{-1}$ where $1\,mmol = 16.1\,g$, so that a haemoglobin concentration of $150\,g \cdot l^{-1}$ would be equivalent to $9.3\,mmol \cdot l^{-1}$. Calculated total CO_2 and plasma HCO_3^- also can be determined by extrapolation of the line.

these values on the nomogram and continued to intersect a line corresponding to the measured haemoglobin concentration in arterial blood. This intersection corresponds to the calculated base excess or base deficit (see page 76). Many blood gas analysers have programmed into them the parameters and equations based on the Siggaard-Andersen nomogram and provide values of base excess and base deficit (as well as a number of other less useful and even more questionable variables). The use of such acid–base nomograms, which are determined from in-vitro equilibration of blood, can lead to errors in the evaluation of acid–base disorders. For example, an increase in PCO_2 to 9.3 kPa (70 mmHg), in the absence of a non-respiratory (metabolic) component, results in a decrease in the pH of the whole body to 7.18. This is a severe but pure respiratory acidosis. However, the Siggaard-Andersen nomogram would predict from these values a component of non-respiratory acidosis with a base deficit of $5 \, mmol \cdot l^{-1}$. This error is reduced if it is assumed that the haemoglobin is distributed throughout the total extracellular fluid compartment. In other words, assume that the haemoglobin concentration is one third the measured value. In practice, the errors involved with the use of in-vitro lines are great only at extremes of acidosis and alkalosis and, as pointed out later in this chapter and again in Chapter 5, treatment of an acid–base disorder should always be by gradual titration back to normal with repeated analyses of blood gas and pH being made. Nevertheless, since the data are available, it is more logical and more accurate for the assessment of acid–base status to be made using in-vivo titration lines.

4.5 Intracellular buffering

A change in the acid–base state of the body is not confined to the blood compartment but rapidly becomes distributed throughout the extracellular fluid. As previously mentioned, this has the effect of decreasing the apparent buffering capacity in the short term but, after a few hours, there is a further and progressive buffering. This is attributed to the effect of intracellular buffers. It has been estimated that, after several hours, about half of an acid load is buffered intracellularly. There is accumulating evidence that the main site of intracellular buffering, particularly in the long term, is in bone (Cogan, Rector & Seldin, 1981). Chronic acidosis leads to demineralisation of bone. Hydrogen ions exchange for sodium, potassium and calcium ions and this leads to the loss of bone solids and frequently to raised levels of plasma potassium. Even after only a few hours of acidosis there is a decrease in bone calcium and carbonate. In one study (Lemann, Litzow & Lennon, 1966), normal subjects were given a high acid load for 18 days. There was a progressive decrease in plasma bicarbonate concentration for 9 days which then remained constant for the remainder of the experimental period despite a continuing positive acid balance. The limit to the change in bicarbonate and pH was attributed mainly to bone buffering. There was a continuous loss of calcium and phosphate. After the end of the period of acidaemia the lost calcium was replaced very slowly and was only partially replaced after several weeks on a normal diet. Buffering by bone is, thus, a possible mechanism whereby individuals with chronic acidosis, such as in renal or metabolic disorders, can maintain a chronic positive acid balance without a fatal change in the pH in the body.

The control and importance of intracellular pH and intracellular buffering to the function of the cell are described in Chapter 3.

4.6 Whole body titration

The response in the body to the addition or removal of carbonic acid and non-volatile or fixed acids can be defined in terms of the effects on the H^+ concentration or pH, the partial pressure of CO_2 and the concentration of HCO_3^-. Usually these variables are determined in samples of arterial blood. Estimates in mixed venous blood, although being related more closely to tissue levels, are less convenient to obtain and do not provide information on the respiratory component. Two simple equations facilitate the understanding of the equilibria:

$$CO_2 + H_2O \rightleftharpoons H_2CO_3 \rightleftharpoons H^+ + HCO_3^- \qquad (4.1)$$

and

$$H^+ + BA^- \rightleftharpoons HBA \qquad (4.2)$$

(BA^- refers to the various buffer anions, mainly haemoglobin in blood; see section 1.3 for further details).

An increase in the level of CO_2 in the blood displaces eqn (4.1) to the right, resulting in increased $[HCO_3^-]$ and increased $[H^+]$. Some of the H^+ ions are buffered by the buffer anions (eqn 4.2) so the concentration of the buffer anions determines the magnitude of the change in pH (see Chapter 1).

An increase in the amount of non-volatile acid, which implies a strong acid which dissociates almost completely to form a large amount of H^+ ions, displaces both equations. Relatively little is buffered by the anions (eqn 4.2). Equation (4.1) is displaced to the left resulting in a decrease in $[HCO_3^-]$. Initially CO_2 is released and the PCO_2 increases. The excess CO_2 is evolved at the lung.

In practice, acid–base balance is readily assessed by the use of blood gas and pH electrode systems (see p. 90). These provide values of PCO_2 and pH only. Since an increase in PCO_2, which is the primary disturbance in a respiratory acidosis, may also occur in a non-respiratory acidosis due to the release of CO_2 (eqn 4.1) when the normal respiratory response is absent, evaluation of the disorder requires a quantitative assessment of the values of pH and PCO_2. Furthermore, an acid–base disorder is rarely simple. For example, a non-respiratory acidosis (retention of non-volatile acid) is likely to be partly compensated for by a respiratory alkalosis. Also a respiratory acidosis (CO_2 retention) may be compensated by a non-respiratory alkalosis due to the renal response (see Chapter 2).

The immediate effects of acid–base disturbances can be studied by use of continuous flow electrode systems. In this way, PCO_2 and pH in an experimental animal are recorded continuously, together with respiratory movements, and the effects of imposed disturbances can be studied.

4.6.1 *Addition of CO_2*
During spontaneous breathing, CO_2 added to the venous blood by a membrane gas exchanger (artificial lung) results in a small increase in PCO_2 and decrease in pH (Figure 4.3a). However, due to the increased respiratory stimulation provided by the CO_2 and H^+ ions, the increase in respiration limits the changes of PCO_2 and pH.

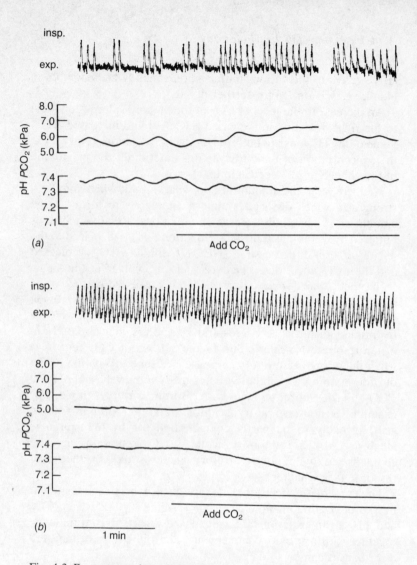

Fig. 4.3 Responses of anaesthetised dog to addition of CO_2 of venous blood by use of a membrane gas exchanger. Records of chest wall movements (respiration) and PCO_2 and pH in arterial blood obtained by continuous flow of arterial blood through electrode systems. CO_2 was added during time shown by horizontal line. (a) Dog breathing spontaneously. Addition of CO_2 resulted in an increase in respiration and relatively small changes PCO_2 and pH. Panel on right, taken in steady state after CO_2 flow at lower level, shows that respiration remained increased although PCO_2 and pH were little changed from the control values. (b) During artificial ventilation, when the respiratory response is prevented, addition of CO_2 resulted in a large increase in arterial PCO_2 and a decrease in pH.

When ventilation is controlled, addition of CO_2 results in a steep increase in arterial PCO_2 and this is mirrored by a decrease in pH (Figure 4.3b). These large changes contrast with the much smaller changes which occur when the respiratory response is able to remove the added CO_2. The same changes can also be obtained in response to a decrease in pulmonary ventilation.

4.6.2 *Addition of non-volatile acid*

An infusion of a strong acid results in an increase in H^+ ions and this results in the displacement of CO_2 from HCO_3^- (eqn 4.1). There is, thus, an increase in PCO_2 as well as a decrease in pH (Figure 4.4a). Respiration is stimulated both by the increase in $[H^+]$ and the increase in PCO_2. During prolonged non-respiratory acidaemia an equilibrium is reached in which both pH and PCO_2 are low.

If acid is infused during controlled respiration, PCO_2 increases and remains high until the excess CO_2 is eliminated by the lung (Figure 4.4b). Mixed disorders can be demonstrated when, after infusion of strong acid, changes in PCO_2 are superimposed.

Note the similarity of the effects on pH and PCO_2 of both addition of CO_2 and infusion of acid (Figures 4.3 and 4.4); both interventions increase PCO_2 and decrease pH. It is only by making a careful quantitative assessment of the changes and relating them to *in vivo* titration lines that it is possible to assess the cause of the disturbance and, therefore, the required treatment.

4.6.3 *Addition of bicarbonate*

An increase in plasma $[HCO_3^-]$ results in the removal of H^+ ions to form H_2CO_3 then CO_2 (eqn 4.1). CO_2 is removed at the lung, leading to a non-respiratory alkalosis. During spontaneous ventilation there would be an initial increase in ventilation until the evolved CO_2 was removed. A bolus injection of HCO_3^- during controlled ventilation would result in an initial increase in PCO_2 (which would gradually return to its control value) and a raised pH.

4.6.4 *Titration lines and non-respiratory pH*

A titration line can be determined from the in-vivo relationship between PCO_2 and pH using the procedure outlined in section

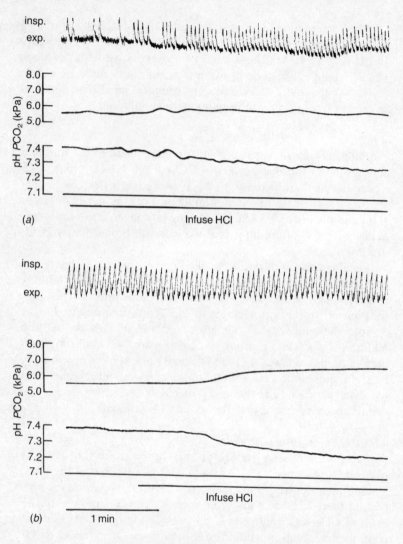

Fig. 4.4 Responses of anaesthetised dog to intravenous infusion of HCl. Preparation and traces as in Fig. 4.3. Infusion of HCl resulted in a decrease in pH and an increase in PCO_2. During spontaneous ventilation (a) the CO_2 released by the acid was evolved at the lung and the change in PCO_2 was small and transient. During artificial ventilation (b), when respiration could not increase, there were much larger changes in pH and PCO_2. Note the **qualititative** similarities of the responses to infusion of acid with the responses to addition of CO_2 (Fig. 4.2).

4.6.1. Different states of non-respiratory acidosis or alkalosis can be induced by adding a strong acid, which removes HCO_3^-, or by infusing $NaHCO_3$ solution, which adds HCO_3^-. The relationship between PCO_2 and pH at each state can, thus, be determined to superimpose a respiratory disturbance over a non-respiratory disturbance. Figure 4.5 shows values of PCO_2 and pH, determined continuously in an anaesthetised dog, following changes in pulmonary ventilation and infusion of HCl. In Figure 4.5*a*, initially PCO_2 was 5.3 kPa and pH was 7.40. Increasing ventilation decreased PCO_2 and increased pH. Then decreases in ventilation increased PCO_2 and decreased pH. Figure 4.5*b* shows records from the same experiment after the infusion of HCl and the adjustment of PCO_2. The value of pH when PCO_2 was 5.3 kPa was about 7.25. The decrease in pH from 7.40 to 7.25 when PCO_2 remained at 5.3 kPa represents a pure non-respiratory acidosis. The effects on PCO_2 and pH were then recorded when ventilation was changed to examine the effects of respiratory alkalosis and acidosis superimposed on the non-respiratory acidosis. These data points can be plotted to obtain a series of CO_2 titration curves at different states of non-respiratory acidaemia. Figure 4.6 was drawn from the data obtained by Kappagoda, Linden & Snow (1970) from anaesthetised dogs and subsequently confirmed in humans (Stoker, Kappagoda, Grimshaw & Linden, 1972). Any point lying on the heavy line represents a pure respiratory disorder; above the PCO_2 value of 5.3 kPa (40 mmHg) there is a respiratory acidosis, below 5.3 kPa, a respiratory alkalosis. Any value of pH when PCO_2 is 5.3 kPa represents a pure non-respiratory disorder. The other lines denote mixed disorders. Any point to the left of the heavy line denotes a mixed disorder with a component of non-respiratory acidosis. The non-respiratory component can be assessed in terms of the **non-respiratory pH**. This is the pH value which would be obtained when PCO_2 is corrected to 5.3 kPa. The dotted lines in Figure 4.5 indicate how the non-respiratory pH is determined.

4.7 **Management of acute acid–base disorders**

Wherever possible, acid–base disorders should be treated as they develop and before they become severe. Frequent assessment of pH and PCO_2 during physiological experiments on anaesthetised

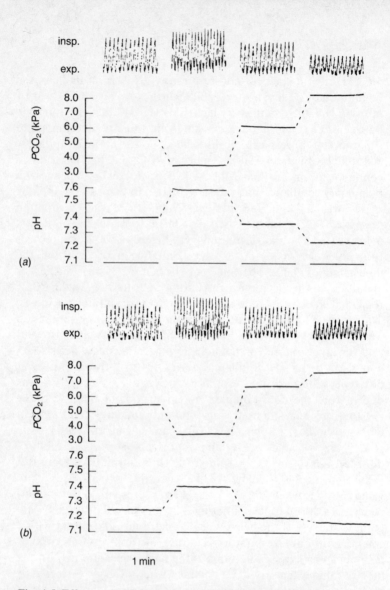

Fig. 4.5 Effects on PCO_2 and pH in anaesthetised dog of changes in ventilation. Traces as in Fig. 4.3. (*a*) Ventilation and acid–base state adjusted in left panel so that PCO_2 and pH were close to 5.3 kPa and 7.40 units. Subsequent panels show the effects of increasing then decreasing ventilation. (*b*) A non-respiratory acidosis was created by the infusion of HCl. Left panel: ventilation was adjusted so that PCO_2 was again 5.3 kPa; i.e. a pure non-respiratory acidosis with pH at 7.25 units. Subsequent panels show effects of changes in ventilation superimposed on the non-respiratory acidosis.

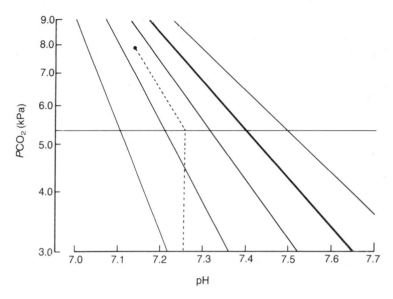

Fig. 4.6 Whole body titration lines. Drawn from data of Kappagoda et al. (1970). Each line was drawn from data of the type shown in Fig. 4.5. To evaluate the non-respiratory component of a disorder the values of pH and PCO_2 are plotted on this diagram and a line drawn along the titration lines to intercept the line of PCO_2 at 5.3 kPa. The corresponding value of pH is the non-respiratory pH and is a measure of the degree of non-respiratory acidosis or alkalosis. The dotted lines illustrate this method of calculation and show that when the values of PCO_2 and pH are 7.8 kPa and 7.13, the non-respiratory pH is 7.26.

animals, during major surgery in humans, and in the management of seriously ill patients, can detect early changes in acid–base state and allow treatment before serious disorders occur. During prolonged experiments on anaesthetised animals there is a tendency for a non-respiratory acidosis to develop and, during spontaneous ventilation, for a respiratory acidosis also. I find that a continuous infusion of $NaHCO_3$ (about $50\,\mu mol \cdot min^{-1} \cdot kg^{-1}$; i.e. $1\,mmol \cdot min^{-1}$ to a 20 kg dog) not only prevents a non-respiratory acidosis, but results in more successful experiments than those performed when an acidosis is allowed by develop and is subsequently treated.

If an acid–base disturbance has developed, as assessed by Figure 4.6, treatment of a respiratory component, where applicable, is by changing the pulmonary ventilation. Treatment of a non-respiratory acidosis is by addition, preferably by slow infusion $(100\,\mu\text{mol}\cdot\text{kg}^{-1}\cdot\text{min}^{-1})$, of $NaHCO_3$. The progress of this titration is monitored by frequent estimations of blood gases and pH and reference to the titration lines (Figure 4.6). Remember that addition of HCO_3^- displaces the equations,

$$CO_2 + H_2O \rightleftharpoons H_2CO_3 \rightleftharpoons H^+ + HCO_3^-,$$

to the left and, unless there is an adequate respiratory response to the increased CO_2, there may be a large increase in PCO_2, particularly if HCO_3^- is given rapidly. When large bolus injections or more rapid infusions of HCO_3^- are given, not only will there be potentially large increases in PCO_2 and pH, but much of the infused HCO_3^- will be lost in the urine and the total amount of HCO_3^- required will be considerably greater than when low infusion rates are used.

Note that the quantitative relationships shown in Figure 4.6 relate to acute changes only. Different relationships may apply in chronic acidaemic states (see Chapter 5). However, the same principles for treatment apply: slowly infuse HCO_3^- and make frequent estimates of pH and PCO_2.

4.8 Estimation of blood pH and PCO_2

These are almost always determined now by use of commercially produced electrode systems. These systems vary in degree of sophistication, but are based on the same principles. Reliable estimates can be obtained only by careful and skilful collection of the sample and use of the apparatus.

4.8.1 *Withdrawal of arterial blood*
Suitable arteries for the withdrawal of blood are the brachial, radial and femoral. In unskilled hands, arterial puncture can be distressing and can lead to changes in breathing and consequent changes in pH and PCO_2. If only a single blood sample is required, a simple needle puncture is generally used. If repeated samples are required, it is preferable to insert a catheter. Whichever is used, a local anaesthetic, e.g. 1 per cent lignocaine **without** adrenaline,

should first be infiltrated. To insert a catheter, the Seldinger technique is used. A sterile Cournand or Riley needle is inserted into the artery. A guide wire is then passed through this needle into the artery and the needle removed. Finally, a catheter is fed over the guide wire into the artery and the guide wire removed. A tap is fitted to the catheter which allows repeated samples to be taken. To ensure that arterial blood is being collected note that the flow of blood from the needle or catheter is pulsatile and is under a high pressure, usually sufficient to push back the barrel of the syringe. The catheter must be left full of heparinised saline.

Blood is collected in a heparinised syringe. Since heparin is an acidic solution, use a dilute solution $(100–500 \, i.u. \cdot ml^{-1})$ and the minimum quantity required to fill the dead space of the syringe. If a catheter is in place, first discard the saline in the catheter using a separate syringe. Slowly withdraw the blood into the syringe, over several respiratory cycles to even out respiratory variations in blood gases and pH, and avoid contamination of the sample with air. If a small air bubble is present, carefully remove this before fitting the syringe with a cap and mixing the blood with the heparin.

Ideally the sample should be analysed immediately. If this is not possible and blood must be stored for longer than a few minutes, the sample should be cooled by placing the syringe in ice. This is because blood is continuously metabolising to decrease the oxygen tension and to increase PCO_2 and decrease pH. At body temperature, PCO_2 and pH change by about $+1 \, kPa \cdot h^{-1}$, and $-0.05 \, units \cdot h^{-1}$ respectively. In ice PCO_2 and pH change by only $+0.2 \, kPa \cdot h^{-1}$ and $-0.01 \, units \cdot h^{-1}$. The effect on the oxygen tension depends on the part of the dissociation curve considered. At body temperature, oxygen content decreases by about $0.5 \, ml \cdot l^{-1} \cdot h^{-1}$ which at high oxygen tensions would lead to a very large change in the tension.

4.8.2 *Electrode systems*

The principles of the pH electrode are shown in Figure 4.7. Blood pH is analysed by use of a glass electrode system. Blood is introduced into a chamber which incorporates special pH sensitive glass. A potential difference occurs across the glass which is proportional to the difference in H^+ concentrations. The potential

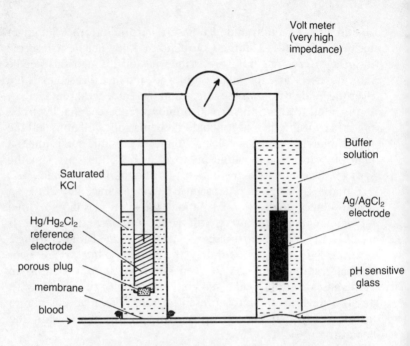

Fig. 4.7 The pH glass electrode system. A potential difference is developed across pH sensitive glass which is a function of the difference in the $[H^+]$ across the glass. The potential difference generated by the pH in the sample is compared with a stable reference electrode system. This system is calibrated by use of buffers of known pH.

difference is compared with that across a very stable Hg/Hg_2Cl_2 (calomel) reference electrode and the circuit completed using a $Ag/AgCl_2$ electrode and a bridge of saturated KCl. The system is calibrated before each use using buffer solutions of known pH.

The PCO_2 electrode (Figure 4.8) is really a modified pH electrode. Instead of pH sensitive glass being in direct contact with the blood, it is separated from it by a membrane, which is permeable to CO_2, and a solution containing $NaHCO_3$. Carbon dioxide diffuses across the membrane and leads to the formation of H^+ ions as shown below:

$$CO_2 + H_2O \rightleftharpoons H_2CO_3 \rightleftharpoons H^+ + HCO_3^-$$

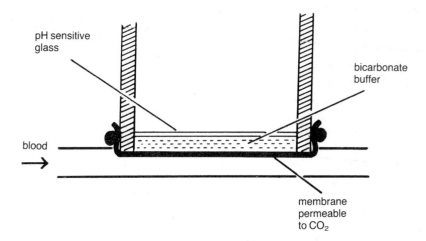

Fig. 4.8 Construction of PCO_2 electrode. In this electrode system, the blood is separated from the glass pH electrode by a thin membrane. CO_2 diffuses readily across this membrane and the carbonic acid dissociates to form H^+ ions. It is these H^+ ions that are estimated by the glass electrode.

Hence,

$$PCO_2 \propto [H^+] \cdot [HCO_3^-] \qquad (4.3)$$

The presence in the solution of HCO_3^- means that small changes in the amount of HCO_3^-, due to changes in PCO_2, have little effect on the total $[HCO_3^-]$ and $[H^+]$ is effectively proportional to PCO_2. The $[H^+]$ in the solution is determined by use of the pH sensitive glass and the electrode assembly. This system is calibrated by use of gases in which the CO_2 tension is known.

Note that the values obtained by use of the electrode systems are dependent on temperature. The electrodes are normally maintained at normal body temperature (37 °C). However, if blood is withdrawn from a subject at a different temperature (hypothermia or fever) there will be a change in the values recorded. It is possible to correct for such temperature shifts by use of appropriate tables (e.g. Adams & Hahn, 1982).

4.9 **Further reading**

Adams, A. P. & Hahn, C. E. W. (1982). *Principles and practice of blood-gas analysis*. 2nd edn. Churchill Livingstone, Edinburgh.

Cogan, M. G., Rector, F. C. & Seldin, D. W. (1981). 'Acid–base disorders.' In: B. M. Brenner & F. C. Rector *The Kidney*. 2nd edn. Saunders, Philadelphia.

Daly, M. de B. & Scott, M. J. (1968). The effects of stimulation of the carotid body chemoreceptors on heart rate in the dog. *J. Physiol.* **144**, 148–66.

Linden, R. J. & Mary, D. A. S. G. (1983). 'The preparation and maintenance of anaesthetized animals for the study of cardiovascular function.' In: *Techniques in the Life Sciences. Physiology*, volume P3/1, *Techniques in Cardiovascular Physiology*, Part 1.

Hainsworth, R., Karim, F., McGregor, K. H. & Wood, L. M. (1983). Responses of abdominal vascular resistance and capacitance to stimulation of carotid chemoreceptors in anaesthetized dogs. *J. Physiol.* **334**, 409–19.

Hainsworth, R., Karim, F. & Sofola, A. O. (1979). Left ventricular inotropic responses to stimulation of carotid body chemoreceptors in anaesthetized dogs. *J. Physiol.* **287**, 455–66.

Hainsworth, R., McGregor, K. H., Rankin, A. J. & Soladoye A. O. (1984). Cardiac inotropic responses from changes in carbon dioxide tension in the cephalic circulation of anaesthetized dogs. *J. Physiol.* **357**, 23–35.

Harry, J. D., Kappagoda, C. T., Linden, R. J. & Snow, H. M. (1971). Depression of the reflex tachycardia from the left atrial receptors by acidaemia. *J. Physiol.* **218**, 465–75.

Kappagoda, C. T., Linden, R. J. & Snow, H. M. (1970). An approach to the problems of acid–base balance. *Clin. Sci.* **39**, 169–82.

Lassen, N. A. (1974). Control of cerebral circulation in health and disease. *Circ. Res.* **34**, 749–60.

Lemann Jr., J., Litzow, J. R. & Lennon, E. J. (1966). The effects of chronic acid loads in normal man: further evidence for the participation of bone mineral in the defense against chronic metabolic acidosis. *J. Clin. Invest.* **45**, 1608–14.

Levesque, P. R. (1975). Acid–base disorders: application of total body carbon dioxide titration in anesthesia. *Anesthes & analges* **54**, 299–307.

Siggaard-Andersen, O. (1962). The pH-log PCO_2 blood acid base nomogram revised. *Scand. J. Clin. & Lab. Invest.* **14**, 598–604.

Stoker, J. B., Kappagoda, C. T., Grimshaw, V. A. & Linden, R. J. (1972). A new method of assessing states of acute acidaemia in man. *Clin. Sci.* **42**, 455–63.

5

Acid-base balance for the clinician

D. C. Flenley Department of Respiratory Medicine, University of Edinburgh

5.1 **Introduction**

Medical students do find acid–base balance difficult to understand, and it seems that part of the reason is the wide divergence of terms used to describe the problems, and the different approaches used by teachers at different phases of the medical course. This chapter is concerned with the understanding of acid–base balance as it is applied in everyday clinical practice to problems at the bedside, particularly from the standpoint of a physician involved in the care of patients with respiratory disorders, both acute and chronic, where recognition and correction of acid–base disturbances are fundamental to understanding how a patient got into a particular clinical state, and how to get him out of it.

5.2 **History**

CO_2 was first discovered in the early seventeenth century in Brussels, but was rediscovered by Joseph Black in Glasgow, as described in his M.D. thesis in 1756. Before leaving the chair of Chemistry in Glasgow for a similar appointment in Edinburgh in 1767, Black showed that CO_2 was involved in human respiration by a grandiose experiment where he placed rags soaked in lime water in the air vent of a Glasgow kirk, where 1 500 people were congregated for ten hours at their religious devotions, thereby generating a 'considerable quantity' of crystallised lime from the reaction of their exhaled CO_2 with the lime water in the rags. Today concepts of biological acid–base chemistry have stemmed largely from Copenhagen, where in 1909 Sorensen described both the electrometric determination of hydrogen ion activity and the pH notation, these methods being applied to the measurement of blood pH by Hasselbalch and Lundsgaard in 1912. In 1917 studies of diabetes in the Rockefeller Institute led Van Slyke to develop his volumetric blood gas apparatus to determine plasma CO_2 concentrations followed in 1924 by the classic description of the manometric apparatus for making this measurement.

Peters and Van Slyke presented a masterly clinical analysis of disturbances of acid–base balance in their 'Quantitative Clinical Chemistry' published in 1931. The principles they enunciated have scarcely changed today. The glass electrode, which today everyone uses to measure pH, was first introduced by MacInnes and Dole in 1929, and was developed most elegantly by Astrup and his colleagues (1956), again in Copenhagen. Their microelectrode allowed them, with interpolation and tonometry, to measure PCO_2 and pH and to calculate base excess in small blood samples. About this time Severinghaus and Bradley (1958) devised the directly reading PCO_2 electrode. Today we have a wide range of automated instruments which measure PCO_2 and pH as well as PO_2 in blood and other body fluids, in microlitre samples. Thus, blood acid–base measurements have become an everyday part of clinical medicine, a far cry from the first recognition of a medical acid–base disorder, which was attributable to O'Shaughnessy, in a description of Asiatic cholera seen in Newcastle, in a letter to the Lancet in 1831. He noted a deficiency of 'carbonate of soda' in the blood of his patients with cholera. This description of metabolic (or non-respiratory) acidosis (as we would now call it), led Latta to the successful use of alkaline salt water injections in the treatment of cholera in the following year.

5.3 Acids and bases

An acid is defined as a proton donor, and a base is a proton acceptor. In water, its uniquely high dielectric constant causes ionic dissociation of an acid. Although the resultant solution probably contains very few free protons, this proton activity generates an electromotive fòrce (e.m.f.) in a hydrogen electrode in contact with the solution. Colloquially this e.m.f. is regarded as being related to the hydrogen ion (H^+) concentration, but thermodynamic theory recognises that the conditions for an ideal solution, where each component of the solution is unaffected by any other, can never be attained in practice.

Thus, the e.m.f. of the free protons in the solution is a function of H^+ **activity** which is related to H^+ **concentration** ($[H^+]$) by the activity coefficient. The biological properties of acids are also related to their $[H^+]$ and it is this which is measured by the pH electrode, so that pH measurements can assess acid–base balance in clinical practice.

Sorensen defined pH as

$$pH = \log\frac{1}{[H^+]} = -\log[H^+] \tag{5.1}$$

Proton acceptors exactly balance proton donors at pH 7.0, when $[H^+]$ is $100\,\text{nmol}\cdot l^{-1}$. In man, a pH range of 6.5–7.7 ($[H^+]$ from $250\,\text{nmol}\cdot l^{-1}$ to $18\,\text{nmol}\cdot l^{-1}$) covers the range of values which appear to be compatible with life. In health the arterial blood has a pH of 7.36–7.44 ($[H^+]$ of $44–36\,\text{nmol}\cdot l^{-1}$).

5.4 **Buffers** (see section 1.2)

Strong acids (e.g. hydrochloric acid, sulphuric acid) are fully dissociated in water, whereas weak acids (e.g. carbonic acid, lactic acid) are only partly dissociated, to an extent which is defined by their dissociation constant (K). K is usually expressed as a logarithm in line with the pH notation

$$pK = \log\frac{1}{K} = -\log K \tag{5.2}$$

The most important buffer in human plasma is the bicarbonate system

$$H_2CO_3 \rightleftharpoons H^+ + HCO_3^- \tag{5.3}$$

with a pK of 6.1. Another important buffer is the phosphate system

$$H_2PO_4^- \rightleftharpoons H^+ + HPO_4^{2-} \tag{5.4}$$

with a pK of 6.8. However, the carboxyl and amino groups of plasma proteins are also very important buffers in blood, and in the red cell by far the most important buffer is the haemoglobin molecule. The bicarbonate buffer system is unique, for the formation of carbonic acid (H_2CO_3) arises from the reversible reaction of CO_2 in solution with water. This reaction is catalysed by carbonic anhydrase (c.a.) which is present in the red cell, renal tubules and gastric mucosa, and also probably in the pulmonary capillary endothelium. The resultant equation

$$\underset{\underset{\text{c.a.}}{\downarrow}}{} CO_2 + H_2O \rightleftharpoons \underset{\underset{\substack{\text{ionic} \\ \text{dissociation}}}{\downarrow}}{} H_2CO_3 \rightleftharpoons H^+ + HCO_3^- \qquad (5.5)$$

is the key to human acid–base balance, as its components are present in plasma, red cells, tissue fluids, cerebrospinal fluid (c.s.f.), urine and also within cells. Hydrogen ions generated or lost in the activation of this equation are interchangeable with H^+ in any other body buffer system in that particular compartment, and this **isohydric principle** means that a description of the acid–base status based on the bicarbonate buffer system will also describe the H^+ changes resulting from all other buffer systems in that compartment of body fluid. It is important to note here that intracellular [H^+] is very different from that in the extracellular fluid, and varies a little from cell to cell. Human red blood cells have an intracellular pH of around 7.20, when blood pH is 7.40 and PCO_2 5.3 kPa (40 mmHg). Human muscle cells (the most abundant tissue in the body) when resting, have an intracellular pH of 6.8–7.0, but as lactic acid is produced by muscular contraction, human muscle intracellular pH falls towards 6.4. Cerebrospinal fluid has a pH of around 7.32 when plasma pH is around 7.4 and, as the protein level of c.s.f. is very low, HCO_3^- is its most important buffer, so that PCO_2 affects the [H^+] of c.s.f. very much.

In clinical practice, however, the acid–base status of the body is best assessed by examination of the blood, either arterial blood, where measurements of pH, PCO_2 and PO_2 are part of everyday clinical practice, or venous blood, where [HCO_3^-] is usually included in standard measurements of serum electrolytes.

5.5 **The acid–base diagram**

Applying the law of mass action to the first dissociation of carbonic acid, given in eqn (5.5), yields

$$[H^+] = K\frac{[CO_2]}{[HCO_3^-]} \qquad (5.6)$$

This can be related to CO_2 in the gas phase (PCO_2) by

$$[H^+] = K\frac{\alpha PCO_2}{[HCO_3^-]} \qquad (5.7)$$

where α is the solubility coefficient of CO_2. Equation (5.7) indicates that PCO_2 can be plotted against arterial $[H^+]$ (expressed in $nmol \cdot l^{-1}$) on linear, non-logarithmic scales, in which straight line isopleths of constant $[HCO_3^-]$ radiate from the origin. Alternatively, if the pH notation is preferred this can also be included on the diagram (Figure 5.1).

Changes in acid–base balance which primarily arise from alterations in PCO_2 are defined as **respiratory acid–base disturbances**, whereas those in which the bicarbonate component (HCO_3^-) is primarily disturbed are defined as non-respiratory components or **metabolic acid–base disturbances**. Definition of any two components of the three part system (molecular CO_2 in solution, H^+ and HCO_3^-) means that there can only be a unique value for the third. The non-respiratory component has been described by various terms, including **base excess**, which is defined as the amount of base required to titrate a blood sample to pH 7.40 and arterial PCO_2 of 5.3 kPa (40 mmHg) at 38 °C. This term base excess has now replaced the older term **standard bicarbonate** which was defined as the $[HCO_3^-]$ of whole blood when this had been equilibrated with a PCO_2 of 5.3 kPa (40 mmHg) at 38 °C. These measurements are independent of the PCO_2, and thus imply that the non-respiratory component will not change as the PCO_2 rises in the blood in life, within the body. In the body this is **not true**, because although the extravascular buffers in body fluids contain no red cells with haemoglobin, as the PCO_2 of body tissues rises hydrogen ions diffuse from extravascular tissues into the blood which **does** have these powerful additional buffers. How-

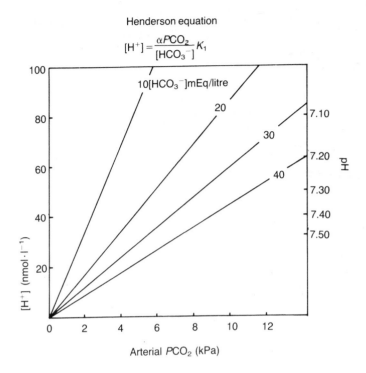

Fig. 5.1 Graphic representation of the Henderson equation relating the acidity ([H^+] in $nmol \cdot l^{-1}$ or pH) of arterial blood to PCO_2 with straight line isopleths of constant [HCO_3^-] radiating from the origin.

ever, if CO_2 is added to blood in a test tube this transfer of CO_2 to poorly buffered body fluids cannot occur, and then the non-respiratory measurements do remain constant. *The non-respiratory pH* (see Chapter 4) is derived from whole body titration curves and is the pH in the blood which would occur when arterial PCO_2 was adjusted to 5.3 KPa.

However, this distinction between what happens to the blood outside the body and to blood within the body is of no real relevance in clinical medicine; it has merely served to distract physiologists and greatly confuse medical students. The debate about this distinction became known as the 'Great trans-Atlantic acid–base debate' (Bunker, 1965) which clinicians have finally decided has been won by the Boston side. This clinician adheres strongly to this view, and in the rest of this discussion acid–base balance, for clinical purposes, will depend upon use of **whole body CO_2 titration curves**, as defined empirically in the arterial blood of whole human beings in life! This position requires no apology for, as in many other systems of medicine, the empirical description of acid–base disturbances (as seen in carefully defined single disease states) allows interpretation which is valuable in diagnosis and guides therapy in practice. The methods used to measure the primary variables, PCO_2 and pH (or $[H^+]$) in arterial blood are irrelevant. It is true that the interpolation method of Astrup (which has been widely used by Siggaard-Anderson (1964) in conjunction with his nonogram), depending upon the equilibration of an arterial blood sample with gases of two known values of PCO_2, and measurement of the pH of these blood samples after equilibration, is a perfectly valid way of arriving at the PCO_2 of the actual blood sample, at the actual pH that is measured when the blood is first taken anaerobically from the body. However, one important methodological point must be stressed. These measurements must be made at body temperature, on blood which has been taken from the artery anaerobically, and then stored anaerobically for no longer than five minutes after leaving the body (see also chapter 4). Thus, the ideal place for any blood-gas machine is in the ward or intensive care unit where the patient is being looked after, not in some remote laboratory where the blood may become cool, or a long delay may occur before measurements can be made. In skilled hands, which should be those of every doctor practising in hospital, arterial puncture to obtain such an anaerobic sample of arterial blood is simple, safe and painless, provided that local anaesthetic is always infiltrated around the left brachial artery, which is the preferred site of puncture. Skill in arterial puncture should be gained by any house physician or house surgeon during his pre-registration house officer appointments in hospital, if not before qualification, in his hospital apprenticeship years.

5.6 Respiratory acid–base disturbances

Here the major problem is either retention of CO_2, with a resultant raised arterial PCO_2, or over-breathing, for whatever

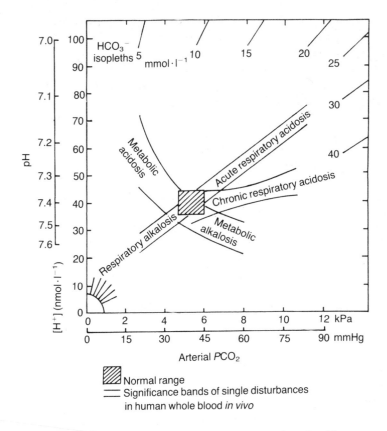

Fig. 5.2 Acid–base diagram of arterial blood showing the 95 per cent confidence limits of the $[H^+]/PCO_2$ relationship for acute and chronic respiratory acidosis *in vivo*, with linear extrapolation of the acute band to include respiratory alkalosis and the significance bands for *in vivo* metabolic acidosis and alkalosis. The shaded area defines the normal range.

cause, resulting in a low arterial PCO_2. If normal healthy subjects are given CO_2 to breathe, and their arterial blood is sampled when the inspired CO_2 is held constant over periods of several minutes, the relationship between PCO_2 and pH (or $[H^+]$) in their arterial blood is defined by the band marked 'acute respiratory acidosis' on Figure 5.2. If, however, such CO_2 inhalation is continued for several days, an experiment which has never been carried out in man but has been studied in dogs, then the renal tubules re-absorb HCO_3^-, increasing the $[HCO_3^-]$ in the plasma and increasing the buffering power of the blood, so that the pH falls although the PCO_2 remains high. The pH/PCO_2 relationships in arterial blood now lie within the 'chronic respiratory acidosis' band of Figure 5.2. Many studies of patients with chronic CO_2 retention from lung disease (e.g. chronic bronchitis and emphysema, cystic fibrosis, etc.), who were not receiving diuretics or other drugs that may affect acid–base balance, show $[H^+]$/PCO_2 relationships which lie within this significance band for chronic respiratory acidosis.

In contrast, when the primary disturbance is hyperventilation, arterial PCO_2 is reduced. This occurs characteristically in patients with acute pneumonia, pulmonary oedema, bronchial asthma etc., and almost certainly arises from stimulation of vagal afferent fibres within the lungs, because (at least in animal studies) elegant experiments have shown that vagal blockade can prevent hyper-ventilation. Many medical students (and some of their teachers) think that the hyperventilation in these conditions is due to the concomitant hypoxia which arises, but clinical experience shows that administering oxygen to these patients can correct the arterial hypoxaemia but does not restore the PCO_2 to normal. Thus, the hypoxaemia seen in patients with pneumonia, pulmonary oedema, bronchial asthma etc. contributes very little to the excessive ventilation (shown by a low PCO_2) of these patients. However, in the high altitude much loved by physiologists, hypoxia is indeed the primary stimulus to the hyperventilation which reduces the PCO_2. In this circumstance, as in the clinical conditions dis-cussed above, the patient suffers from respiratory alkalosis, with $[H^+]$/PCO_2 relationships lying within the significance band of 'respiratory alkalosis' shown on Figure 5.2.

An important teaching point is now revealed. Looking at Figure 5.2 it is obvious that one could draw an isopleth of $[HCO_3^-]$ radiating from the origin at a level between 25 and $30 \, nmol \cdot l^{-1}$ (pretty well the normal value) which would encompass the whole range of values of PCO_2, from the most severe respiratory alkalosis known to be compatible with life, to the most severe acute respiratory acidosis. This clearly reveals that **measurement of the $[HCO_3^-]$ alone is not an adequate description of acid–base balance in respiratory disturbances.**

5.7 Metabolic acid–base disturbances

The primary abnormality in metabolic acid–base disturbances is either a change in $[H^+]$ or a change in $[HCO_3^-]$. This contrasts with respiratory disorders where a change in PCO_2 is the primary abnormality.

Metabolic acidosis causes an increase in ventilation, stimulated by the rise in arterial $[H^+]$ acting on the central chemoreceptors mediated through the c.s.f., and via the peripheral carotid and aortic chemoreceptors. The 95 per cent confidence limits for metabolic acidosis shown in Figure 5.2 were derived from patients with untreated diabetic ketoacidosis (Fulop, Dreyer & Tanner baum, 1974; Fulop, 1976), chronic stable renal failure (Cowie, Lambie & Robson, 1962; Albert, Bell & Winters, 1967), and untreated cholera (Pierce *et al.*, 1970). Similar relationships were obtained from patients undergoing repeated haemodialysis (Lambie, Anderton & Cowie, 1965) for chronic renal failure. In clinical practice the severity of metabolic acidosis can often be assessed by $[HCO_3^-]$ values alone, usually by measuring this value in venous blood. Figure 5.2 shows why this is so useful: if one is certain on clinical grounds that the acidosis is only of metabolic origin then, as the significance band of arterial $[H^+]/PCO_2$ values cross the HCO_3^- isopleths at almost right angles, it is obvious that measuring $[HCO_3^-]$ alone will define a close range of arterial $[H^+]/PCO_2$ values and, thus, define the severity of the metabolic acidosis with some accuracy.

Metabolic alkalosis had been defined as a blood $[H^+]$ which is lower than that which would be predicted for the prevailing PCO_2 (Coe, 1977), based upon the significance bands for acute respiratory acidosis and respiratory alkalosis. This definition would imply that any value lying in the chronic respiratory acidosis band indicated a metabolic alkalosis. I think this merely causes confusion so I reject the definition offered by Coe. I prefer a definition based upon clinical, physiological and biochemical findings, because patients with chronic respiratory acidosis can then be eliminated by including in the definition of metabolic alkalosis a requirement that the patient's respiratory function is normal.

By this definition accepted causes of metabolic alkalosis include loss of gastric juice due to high upper intestinal obstruction or nasogastric suction (e.g. in pyloric stenosis), the use of diuretics (thiazides, frusemides and ethacrynic acid) and, of course, administration of large doses of either absorbable alkali orally, or intravenous bicarbonate. In these conditions the urinary chloride concentration is usually low, there is also a less common group of disorders causing metabolic alkalosis in which the urinary chloride level is high. These disorders include hyperaldosteronism, Bartter's syndrome (hyperplasia of the granular cells of the juxtaglomerular apparatus of the kidney with associated renal potassium wasting, normotension, and hyporesponsiveness of arterial blood pressure to infused angiotensin II), Cushing's syndrome (excessive production of cortisol by the adrenal glands due to bilateral adrenal hyperplasia, non-endocrine tumours secreting biologically active polypeptides which are biologically indistinguishable from ACTH, or tumours of the adrenal glands), ingestion of liquorice and, most commonly, severe and prolonged potassium deficiency. In profound metabolic alkalosis there is usually severe reduction in the volume of the extracellular fluid, so that renal function is impaired, which often compounds the potassium depletion. Correction of this reduced extracellular fluid volume, and of both the hypokalaemia and the chloride losses are very important in reversing most cases of metabolis alkalosis (Kassirer, 1974; Coe, 1977).

Although it seems reasonable to expect PCO_2 to rise as arterial $[H^+]$ falls, since this would be expected to remove a drive to breathing, in clinical practice the rise in PCO_2 is rarely significant. An arterial $[H^+]$ below $30 \, nmol \cdot l^{-1}$ (pH 7.52) rarely arises in practice, and the width of this curvilinear significance band indicates that even in such cases the PCO_2 will still usually be normal (Tuller & Mehdi, 1971). However, severe metabolic alkalosis may threaten life, interacting with potassium deficiency and hypokalaemia to affect cardiac function by generating arrythmias. If alkalosis persists despite a normal extracellular fluid volume and normal potassium concentration, then acetazolamide (a potent inhibitor of carbonic anhydrase, producing metabolic acidosis), may be necessary. If this fails, direct infusion of hydrochloric acid (Worthley, 1977) (Figure 5.3) may be indicated.

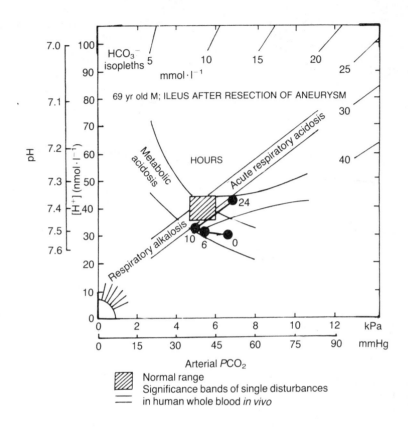

Fig. 5.3 Arterial $[H^+]/PCO_2$ relationships in a 69 year-old man suffering from severe metabolic alkalosis at time 0 hours following development of an ileus, necessitating upper gastro-intestinal suction, after resection of an aortic aneurysm. The sequential values at 6, 10 and 24 hours after intravenous infusion of hydrogen chloride (240 nmol) are shown.

5.8 Clinical examples of the use of the acid–base diagram

A 16-year-old schoolgirl was admitted to hospital with a profound attack of severe asthma, which had increased in severity over two days and had become refractory to inhaled Salbutamol (a β_2 adrenoceptor agonist bronchodilator) and intravenous Amino-

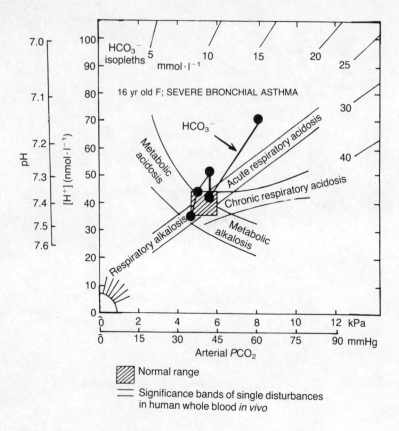

Fig. 5.4 Sequential arterial $[H^+]/PCO_2$ relationships in a 16-year-old asthmatic admitted with CO_2 retention.

phylline (a xanthine bronchodilator). On admission to hospital she was centrally cyanosed, barely rousable, had marked wheeze, indrawing of intercostal spaces, a tachycardia and pulsus paradoxus (a marked inspiratory/expiratory swing in arterial blood pressure). Analysis of arterial blood showed that she had severe CO_2 retention, with a high PCO_2, severe hypoxaemia, and acute respiratory acidosis (Figure 5.4), although on breathing oxygen at $2 1 \cdot min^{-1}$ through nasal prongs her arterial PO_2 rose to $12\,kPa$ ($90\,mmHg$). Prompt treatment with large doses of intravenous corticosteroids, and wet nebulised Salbutamol delivered by a Wright's nebuliser, combined with intravenous HCO_3^- restored her acid–base status towards normal over several hours, but the possibility that mechanical ventilation would be required was always present during this period.

In most cases of severe asthma arterial PCO_2 tends to be normal or low (Figure 5.5), only rising to higher than normal levels in very severe asthma, where the FEV_1 (a simple measure of the limitation to airflow) is reduced to below 20–30 per cent of the predicted normal value for a person of that age and sex. However, although this low PCO_2 is associated with hypoxia, it is not caused by the hypoxia, as correction of arterial hypoxaemia by administration of oxygen does not restore the PCO_2 to normal.

Experimental data in dogs with an experimentally induced allergic asthma shows that cooling of the vagi prevents such hyperventilation with a low PCO_2 in the asthmatic attack, indicating that afferent discharges from the lungs, running within the vagus, are responsible for the primary hyperventilation with a low PCO_2 which is seen in acute asthma. Similar phenomena develop in acute pneumonia, and are probably also the cause of the hyperventilation of pulmonary oedema, from excitation of J receptors whose afferent fibres run in the vagi.

A 58-year-old miner with acute pneumonia due to *Streptococcus pneumoniae* infection was admitted to hospital (day 0) with severe arterial hypoxaemia, but no CO_2 retention. It appeared from his history that he also had chronic bronchitis and emphysema, with a low FEV_1 (indicating airflow limitation). Despite controlled oxygen therapy to relieve some of his hypoxaemia (oxygen given in a dose of $2 \, l \cdot min^{-1}$ by nasal prongs), his arterial PCO_2 rose, so that 1½ days after admission he had a PCO_2 of 19 kPa (75 mmHg) and $[H^+]$ of 70 nmol $\cdot l^{-1}$ (pH 7.15), and was gravely ill (Figure 5.6). In addition to antibiotics to control his pneumonia, he was then given the rather old-fashioned ventilatory stimulant Nikethamide intravenously (today Doxapram would have been used) and this caused a fall in PCO_2 by the second day, with subsequent change back to normal values on the sixth day following hospital admission, as his pneumonia was controlled with the antibiotic therapy. It is noteworthy that these acute changes over the first two days occurred more or less within the

Relationship between P_aCO_2 and $FEV_{1.0}$ in asthma

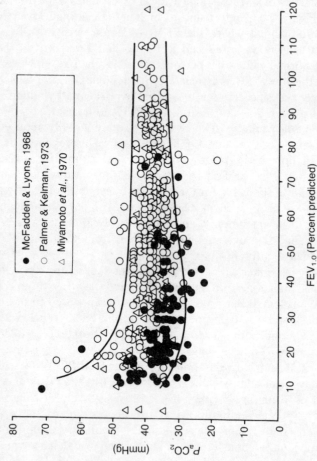

Fig. 5.5 Relationship between $FEV_{1.0}$ (expressed as a percentage of the predicted normal value) and arterial PCO_2 (P_aCO_2) in stable and acute asthma. Mild to moderately severe asthma ($FEV_{1.0}$ 30–70 per cent predicted) is associated with low or normal PCO_2 with hyper-capnia occurring only in severe acute asthma ($FEV_{1.0} < 20$–30 per cent predicted).

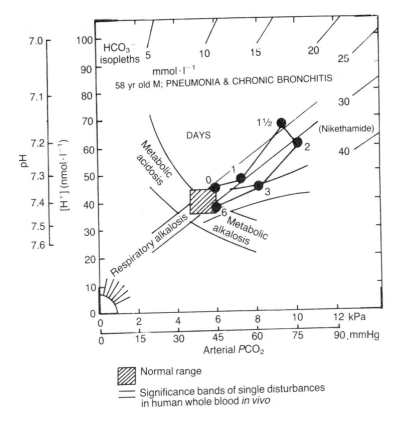

Fig. 5.6 Sequential arterial $[H^+]/PCO_2$ relationships in a 58-year-old man with chronic bronchitis and pneumonia over a period of 6 days from admission.

significance bands of acute respiratory acidosis disturbances, as there was little time for renal tubular reabsorption of HCO_3^- to cause an increase in $[HCO_3^-]$ over this acute period.

A 62-year-old man with severe chronic bronchitis and emphysema was admitted with an exacerbation of his condition, due to a combined respiratory infection with *Haemophilus influenzae* and *Streptococcus pneumoniae*. He was then profoundly hypoxic, with central cyanosis, and the signs of hyperinflation of the chest: indrawing of intercostal spaces, shortening of the

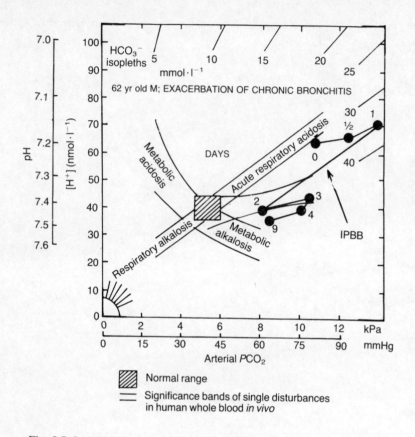

Fig. 5.7 Sequential arterial $[H^+]/PCO_2$ relationships in a 62-year-old man with an acute exacerbation of chronic bronchitis over a period of 9 days from admission.

crico-sternal distance, absence of absolute cardiac dullness, and widening of the subcostal angle. At this time he had elevation of jugular venous pressure and a trace of ankle oedema, indicating that he was probably suffering also from cor pulmonale or right heart failure due to his primary lung disease. He gave a history of chronic cough and spit, with increasing breathlessness, but this history was difficult to obtain as he was very drowsy at the time of his acute admission (day 0: Figure 5.7). Arterial blood-gas analysis then showed that he had a severe hypoxaemia, along with CO_2

retention, and relatively profound respiratory acidosis, with values lying just at the lower level of the acute respiratory band. He was again treated with controlled oxygen therapy (initially $21 \cdot min^{-1}$ by nasal prongs) to try to prevent death from this severe hypoxia. As a result, however, his PCO_2 rose, so that after 24 hours in the hospital his PCO_2 was almost 13 kPa (100 mmHg) when breathing oxygen, with a $[H^+]$ of nearly $70 \, nmol \cdot l^{-1}$ (pH 7.15). Experience has shown that such patients have a grave risk to life when their $[H^+]$ rises above $55 \, nmol \cdot l^{-1}$ during controlled oxygen therapy (Figure 5.8), so he was treated with endotracheal intubation, and intermittent positive pressure breathing (IPBB) with a mechanical ventilator, which reduced his PCO_2 acutely, as shown in Figure 5.7. This was associated with a relative fall in $[H^+]$ and, when ventilation was stopped after 48 hours, his PCO_2 rose a little, but by this time his kidneys had re-absorbed bicarbonate, so that his subsequent values of acid–base variables on days 3, 4 and 9 of his hospital admission lay near to the chronic respiratory acidosis band. Note that the acute change in $[H^+]/PCO_2$ relationships occasioned by mechanical ventilation caused a change which was parallel to the acute respiratory band, as these changes occurred acutely.

A 17-year-old diabetic was admitted to hospital with keto-acidosis, classic Kussmaul's breathing (hissing hyperventilation), severe acidosis, and a low arterial PCO_2.

Diabetic ketoacidosis was corrected by bolus doses of intra-venous and intramuscular insulin (this being in the days before continuous infusion of insulin was practised), combined with large volumes of intravenous saline, but without intravenous bicar-bonate. The serial acid–base data (Figure 5.9) shows values of arterial $[H^+]/PCO_2$ relationships which fell within the metabolic acidosis band initially, and these declined within this band, except for the value at 24 hours after hospital admission, which showed some persistent hyperventilation with a low PCO_2. Although not proven, it seems possible that this could have arisen from persistent acidosis within the cerebrospinal fluid driving ven-tilation at this time. This patient, therefore, suffered from an almost pure metabolic acidosis.

A 48-year-old man was admitted to hospital with small pupils, semi-conscious, and with flecks of blood-stained foam about his

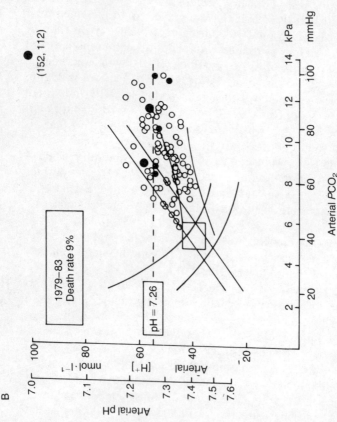

Fig. 5.8 Arterial $[H^+]/PCO_2$ relationship at the time of highest arterial $[H^+]$ (lowest pH) in patients admitted with an acute exacerbation of chronic bronchitis and emphysema treated with controlled oxygen therapy (patients surviving ○; patients dying ●). In patients studied between 1970 and 1976 (A; Warren et al., 1980) the risk of death was found to be significantly higher if $[H^+]$ rose above $55 \, nmol \cdot l^{-1}$ (pH falling below 7.26). This was confirmed in studies of admissions between 1979 and 1983 where the smaller number of

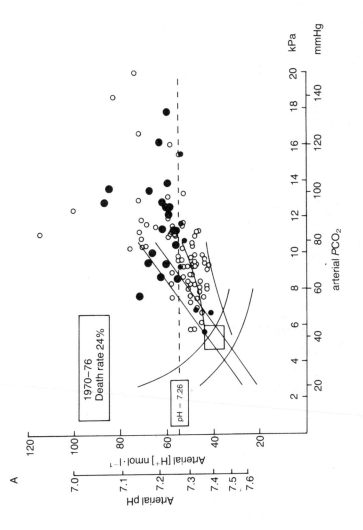

A

1970–76
Death rate 24%

pH = 7.26

arterial PCO₂

Arterial [H⁺] nmol·l⁻¹

Arterial pH

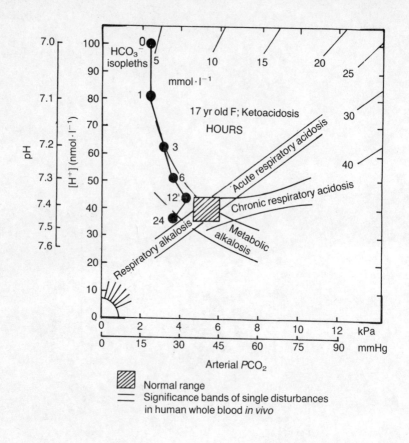

Fig. 5.9 Sequential arterial $[H^+]/PCO_2$ relationships in a 17-year-old diabetic admitted with ketoacidosis over 24 hours following admission.

lips. He was correctly diagnosed as having heroin induced pulmonary oedema and, on analysis of the arterial blood, he was found to have severe CO_2 retention, with very severe acidosis. In fact, $[H^+]$ was greater than could be accounted for on the basis of his retention of CO_2 alone. Thus, he also had an additional lactic acidosis, no doubt due to tissue hypoxia from his low cardiac output coupled with severe arterial hypoxaemia due to the pulmonary oedema. He was initially treated by mechanical

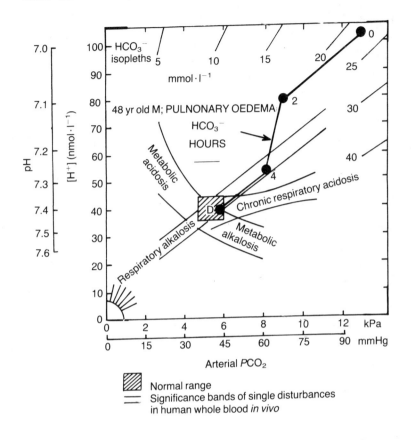

Fig. 5.10 Sequential arterial $[H^+]/PCO_2$ relationships in a 48-year-old man admitted with pulmonary oedema.

ventilation via a cuffed endotracheal tube, and this lowered his PCO_2 but still left him with a $[H^+]$ which was higher than that attributable to the level of PCO_2 alone, as indicated by the acute respiratory acidosis band of Figure 5.10. Therefore, intravenous bicarbonate was given and four hours after hospital admission he had values of acid–base balance which were within the acute respiratory acidosis band. Further improvement of his pulmonary oedema, with response to diuretic therapy and improvement in cardiac output, left him with normal acid–base variables at the time of his discharge from hospital. This case, described by Anthonisen & Smith (1965) is an example of a complicated acid–base disorder.

These examples, all drawn from actual clinical practice, illustrate the value of the $[H^+]/PCO_2$ plot in defining the status of an acid–base disturbance, indicating its severity, and deriving a logical means to treat it. They further emphasise that in clinical practice it is not possible to prescribe a safe and effective treatment of a given degree of acid–base disturbance from one measurement alone, but that sequential measurements of arterial $[H^+]/PCO_2$ relationships are essential during the management of such conditions in order to restore normal function. Thus, the practice of calculating the amount of intravenous bicarbonate (nmol) to be administered by taking the 'base excess' $\times$ 0.3 $\times$ body weight, and expecting that this will correct any metabolic component of an acid–base disturbance is, in fact, fraught with hazard. It is far more useful in practice to administer, say, one half or one quarter of this calculated dose, then repeat the acid–base measurements and titrate the patient individually towards correction of his acid–base disturbance.

5.9 **Further reading**

Albert, M. S., Bell, D. B. & Winters, R. W. (1967). Quantitative displacement of acid–base equilibrium in metabolic acidosis. *Ann. Int. Med.* **66**, 312–22.

Anthonisen, N. R. & Smith, H. J. (1965). Respiratory acidosis as a consequence of pulmonary oedema. *Ann. Intern. Med.* **62**, 991–9.

Astrup, P. (1956). A simple electrometric technique for the determination of carbon-dioxide tensions in blood and plasma, total content of carbon-dioxide in plasma, and bicarbonate content in 'separated' plasma at a fixed carbon-dioxide tension (40 mmHg). *Scand. J. Clin. Lab. Invest.* **8**, 33–43.

Bunker, J. P. (1965). The great trans-Atlantic acid–base debate. *Anesthesiology* **26**, 591–4.

Coe, F. L. (1977). Metabolic alkalosis. *J. Amer. Med. Assoc.* **238**, 2288–90.

Cowie, J., Lambie, A. T. & Robson, J. S. (1962). The influence of extracorporeal dialysis on the acid–base composition of blood and cerebrospinal fluid. *Clin. Sci.* **23**, 397–404.

Flenley, D. C. (1971). Another non-logarithmic acid–base diagram? *Lancet i*, 961–65.

Fulop, M. (1976). The ventilatory response in severe metabolic acidosis. *Clin. Sci. Mol. Med.* **50**, 367–73.

Fulop, M., Dreyer, N. & Tannerbaum, H. (1974). The ventilatory response in diabetic ketoacidosis. *Clin. Sci. Mol. Med.* **46**, 539–49.

Henderson, L. J. (1908). The theory of neutrality regulation in the animal organism. *Am. J. Physiol.* **21**, 427–48.

Hasselbalch, K. A. & Lundsgaard, C. (1912). Electrometrische reaktionbestimmung des blutes bei korpertemperatur. *Bioch. Z.* **38**, 77–91.

Kassirer, J. P. (1974). Serious acid–base disorders. *N. Engl. J. Med.* **291**, 773–6.

Lambie, A. T., Anderton, J. L. & Cowie, J. (1965). Intracellular hydrogen ion concentration in renal acidosis. *Clin. Sci.* **28**, 237–49.

MacFadden, E. R. & Lyons, H. A. (1968). Arterial-blood gas tensions in asthma. *N. Engl. J. Med.* **278**, 1027–32.

MacInnes, D. A. & Dole, M. (1929). Tests of a new type of glass electrode. *Ind. Engng. Chem. Analyt. Edn.* **1**, 57.

Miyamoto, T., Mizuno, K. & Furuya, K. (1970). Arterial blood gases in bronchial asthma. *J. Allergy* **45**, 248–54.

Palmer, K. N. V. & Kelman, G. R. (1975). Pulmonary function in asthmatic patients in remission. *Br. Med. J. i*, 485–6.

Peters, J. P. & Van Slyke, D. D. (1931). *Quantitative Clinical Chemistry* I, p. 912. Williams and Wilkins, Baltimore.

Pierce, N. F., Fedson D. S., Brigham, K. L., Mitra, R. C., Sack, R. B. & Mondal, A. (1970). The ventilatory response to acute base deficit in humans. *Ann. Intern. Med.* **72**, 633–40.

Severinghaus, J. W. & Bradley, A. F. (1958). Electrodes for blood PO_2 and PCO_2 determination. *J. Appl. Physiol.* **13**, 515–20.

Siggaard-Anderson, O. (1964). The acid–base status of the blood. 2nd edn. Monksgaard, Copenhagen.

Tuller, M. A. & Medhi, F. (1971). Compensatory hypoventilation and hypercapnia in primary metabolic alkalosis. *Amer. J. Med.*

50, 281–90.

Van Slyke, D. D. (1917). Studies of acidosis II. A method for the determination of carbon dioxide and carbonates in solution. *J. Biol. Chem.* **30**, 347–68.

Van Slyke, D. D. & Neill, J. M. (1924). The determination of gases in blood and other solutions by vacuum extraction and manometric measurement. *J. Biol. Chem.* **61**, 523–73.

Warren, P. M., Flenley, D. C., Millar, J. S. & Avery, A. (1980) Respiratory failure revisited: acute exacerbations of chronic bronchitis between 1961–68 and 1970–76. *Lancet i*, 467–71.

Worthley, L. I. G. (1977). The rational use of i.v. hydrochloric acid in the treatment of metabolic acidosis. *Br. J. Anaesth.* **49**, 811–17.

Appendix 1

Teaching material on acid–base balance

Film

In the balance. 16 mm colour, sound, 15 min.

J. C. Edwards and M. Moles.

Department of Teaching Media, University of Southampton. For Wessex Regional Health Authority (Sponsor: Janssen Pharmaceuticals).

Distributor: Rank Aldis Training Films & Video 1978
                  P.O. Box. 70,
                  Great West Road,
                  Brentford,
                  Middlesex TW8 9HR.
                  Tel. 01-569 922

Shows the two most commonly occurring acid–base disturbances: respiratory and metabolic acidosis. Respiratory acidosis is shown in a patient who has a flail chest after a motor accident and metabolic acidosis is shown in a patient who has had a cardiac arrest. The chemistry is explained using simple animation and the treatment of these two forms of acid–base disturbances is demonstrated. Other acid–base balance disturbances are mentioned but no attempt is made at an advanced academic treatment of the subject.

Videotape

Whole body buffering in acid-base balance 28 mm colour.

R. Hainsworth.

Department of Cardiovascular Studies, University of Leeds.

Standard U-matic PAL. Copies available on most standard formats.

Distributor: Audiovisual Service,
           University of Leeds,
           Leeds LS2 9JT.
           Tel. 0532 431751.

Shows continuous traces of arterial pH and PCO_2 in anaesthetised dog. Effects shown of adding CO_2 and acid during spontaneous ventilation and artificial ventilation. Whole body titration curves obtained by changing PCO_2 from normal acid–base states then creating non-respiratory acidaemia and again changing PCO_2.

Audiotapes and booklets

Acid–base balance 1 and 2

N. Saunders.

Distributor: BLAT Centre for Health and Medical Education,
           British Medical Association,
           B.M.A. House,
           Tavistock Square,
           London WC1H 9JP.

Audiotapes and booklets for self-instruction; also recording scripts.

Acid–base balance 1 (1978) Acids and bases, buffer solution, CO_2 transport in blood.

Acid–base balance 2 (1979) Respiratory regulation of arterial PCO_2, measurement of blood pH and blood gases, renal regulation of pH, abnormal conditions of blood and tissue fluid pH, treatment of abnormal conditions of pH.

Appendix 2

Class experiments

pH regulation

Department of Physiology, London Hospital Medical College, London

Introduction

Please **read these instructions carefully** on the day preceding the class.

This experiment is designed to demonstrate the respiratory and renal response to metabolic acidosis and alkalosis. The allocation of students to experiments is designed to ensure that each tutorial group will collectively have carried out the whole experiment but, as the class results will be made available within a few days, you should wait for these results before writing up. Your own data may not lead you to the same conclusions if they are analysed alone.

Experimental design and allocation of subjects

There will be three subject groups, one group (control) receives an oral water load while the other two groups receive an oral water load plus either sodium bicarbonate or ammonium chloride capsules.

There will be three experimenters and up to 8 subjects in each group, working as a unit. Students should be allocated as follows:

Students 1, 2 & 3	Experimenters
Students 4 & 5	Control: drinking water
Students 6, 7 & 11	Metabolic acidosis induced by drinking water plus capsules of NH_4Cl
Students 8, 9 & 10	Metabolic alkalosis induced by drinking water plus capsules of $NaHCO_3$

Preparation

Students numbered 4 onwards should empty their bladders on waking on the morning of the experiment, *noting the time*, and refrain from urinating thereafter until the basal urine sample is collected at the beginning of the class. However, there is no need to restrict food or fluid intake for breakfast.

10.15 a.m. On arrival in the Laboratory, weigh the subjects (in kg).

Experimental procedure

Basal samples of alveolar air and urine are collected (in this order). Further samples will be collected one and two hours later, the time of the first urine collection determining time zero. Immediately after the basal urine collection has been made, subjects begin to ingest their doses:

Students 4 & 5	500 ml water over 30 min.
Students 6, 7 & 11	500 ml water with capsules (each containing 1 g) of NH_4Cl, at a dose of $75 \, mg \cdot kg^{-1}$, over 30 min.
Students 8, 9 & 10	500 ml water with capsules (each containing 1 g) of $NaHCO_3$, at a dose of $160 \, mg \cdot kg^{-1}$, over 30 min.

Because it is essential to collect resting alveolar air samples, experimenters should collect these samples from their subjects **before** the urine is voided, at each sampling time. It is important to insist that the subjects sit **silently** for ten minutes before alveolar air is collected in this experiment or the effect on PCO_2 will not be observed. It is a good idea to allow the subjects to read.

The experimenters should also measure (i) the volume, (ii) the pH and (iii) the Na^+ concentration in each urine sample soon after collection. A fraction of each sample (about 30 ml) is then retained in a labelled sample bottle; excess urine can then be discarded.

In the afternoon, experimenters should measure the titratable acidity and the ammonium ion concentration. From these results, calculate:

(a) titratable acidity excreted ($mmol \cdot h^{-1}$)
(b) ammonium ion excreted ($mmol \cdot h^{-1}$)
(c) total $H^+ + NH_4^+$ excreted (the sum of a + b)

Methods for sodium ion concentration measurement, and the titrations for H^+ or NH_4^+ are explained separately below. Please remember to correct all your units to those required on the data sheet; urine flow is in $l \cdot h^{-1}$, concentrations are in $mmol \cdot l^{-1}$, outputs in $mmol \cdot h^{-1}$. Please enter your data in impeccable handwriting and in exactly the right place on the data sheet which will be presented to the computer operator. The decimal point is already entered for every value; don't over-ride this, use it! Please remember to hand in a copy of results for each student before leaving the class. The experimenters should remember to collect sheets for all their subjects before they leave the laboratory, as not all subjects need to be active in the laboratory during the afternoon. This is important; in all studies involving groups of people, a degree of sloth sets in after an hour or two!

Measurement of Na^+ *concentration and output*
Na^+ concentration in urine is estimated by flame photometry.

Estimation of titratable acidity and ammonium ion in urine

Experimental procedure

1 *Estimation of titratable acidity.* Pipette 10 ml of urine into a beaker. Add 2 g of finely pulverised potassium oxalate to precipitate calcium ions and a few drops of phenolphthalein indicator. Shake the mixture for 1–2 min vigorously and then titrate it with 0.05 M NaOH until a faint, but unmistakable, pink colour remains on further shaking. (This will be orange in yellow urine.) Express the result as $mmol \cdot h^{-1}$.

Do not discard the contents of the flask!

2 *Estimation of Ammonium ion.* In a separate flask, put 5 ml of formalin, add 10 ml of water and two drops of phenolphthalein, and titrate with 0.05 M NaOH to the same end point as above. Add the neutralised formalin to the contents of the flask kept from Procedure 1. Acid is liberated according to the eqn (A2.5) in the Theory section, and the pink colour disappears. Titrate the mixture to the same end point as in Procedure 1, using 0.05 M NaOH, and calculate the additional content of H^+ as NH_4^+, expressed as $mmol \cdot h^{-1}$. Add the two outputs to give the **total acidity**, also as $mmol \cdot h^{-1}$.

If urine flow (uf) is in $l \cdot h^{-1}$ then

$$\text{output} = uf \times 5 \times z \; mmol \cdot h^{-1}$$

where z is the number of ml of 0.05 M NaOH used in the titration.

Theory

Titratable acidity. The traditional account of pH regulation describes two principal buffer systems in urine:

$$HPO_4^{2-} + H^+ \rightleftharpoons H_2PO_4^{-} \tag{A2.1}$$

$$NH_3 + H^+ \rightleftharpoons NH_4^+ \tag{A2.2}$$

The phosphate system has a pK of 6.8. As a glomerular filtrate has a pH of about 7.4, and normal urine a pH of 5–6, phosphate is normally filtered almost entirely in the form HPO_4^{2-}, and is then almost completely converted to the form $H_2PO_4^-$ as it travels down the distal convoluted tubule and the collecting ducts.

The 'titratable acidity' of urine may be determined by titration with standard alkali from the observed pH to blood pH (i.e. pH 7.4) but a good approximation of the acidity may be obtained by titration to the first pink colour of phenolphthalein (approximately pH 8.0).

Ammonium ion. The reaction of ammonia with protons has a pK of 9.2. This means that essentially all the ammonia diffusing from tubule cells into the tubular lumen will accept protons to form the ammonium ion. This would provide a straightforward buffer, if cells produced NH_3 in metabolism. In fact, this is not so; NH_4^+ and HCO_3^- are released during the catabolism of amino acids in the body (particularly in the liver), and in normal conditions most of these ions are consumed, in equimolar amounts, in the production of urea. A small amount of NH_4^+ is normally used in synthesising glutamine from glutamic acid, in a reaction which does not consume HCO_3^-. Glutamine may be metabolised in kidney, and NH_4^+ may pass across the renal tubular cell into the lumen (though it does so as NH_3 and a proton exchanged for Na^+), and this reaction also releases again the glutamate ion.

Before we think about the meaning of urinary ammonium ion excretion, we should consider first the stoichiometry of protein catabolism and the mechanism of ureogenesis.

When proteins are fully catabolised, most amino acids yield one NH_4^+ and one HCO_3^-; some dibasic amino acids (e.g. lysine) yield two NH_4^+ and only one HCO_3^-, while some amino acids with a dicarboxylic acid skeleton (aspartate, glutamate) yield one NH_4^+ and two HCO_3^-. A perfectly neutral, well-averaged protein mixture will produce equimolar amounts of NH_4^+ and HCO_3^-, but there exists the theoretical possibility that one might catabolise proteins selectively, and so produce an imbalance in NH_4^+ and HCO_3^- production (or that the diet may be out of balance in this way). There is no experimental evidence available on this point.

The fate of excess nitrogen is to be excreted, normally mainly as urea, with an appreciable fraction being excreted as NH_4^+.

There are several levels at which one can summarise the stoichiometry of the urea cycle. The simplest equation emphasises its potential for generating acidosis:

$$CO_2 + 2NH_4^+ \rightarrow CO(NH_2)_2 + H_2O + 2H^+ \qquad (A2.3)$$

but in each day's metabolism, about one mole of NH_4^+ is being disposed of through this cycle, together with one mole of HCO_3^-, according to the reaction:

$$2NH_4^+ + 2HCO_3^- \rightarrow CO(NH_2)_2 + CO_2 + 3H_2O \quad (A2.4)$$

and when you look at it like this, it does not affect acid–base balance, because the H^+ produced have titrated the HCO_3^+ which were also produced during amino acid breakdown.

Now we should think again about urinary NH_4^+. If the body becomes acidotic,

(1) NH_4^+ utilisation in the urea cycle is reduced
(2) NH_4^+ utilisation in glutamine synthesis is increased
(3) High levels of glutaminase (the enzyme which releases NH_4^+ again) build up in renal tubular epithelium
(4) The pH of the tubular luminal contents is reduced
(5) The low tubular luminal pH enhances the trapping of NH_4^+ in the primitive urine

(6) The high concentration of NH_4^+ within the cells (due to glutaminase activity) reinforces this process

(7) consequently, NH_4^+ excretion rises; normal urinary NH_4^+ excretion amounts to about $50\,mmol \cdot day^{-1}$, but in prolonged severe acidosis, as much as $500\,mmol \cdot day$ may be excreted.

Given that most proteins yield equal amounts of NH_4^+ and HCO_3^-, the suppression of ureogenesis in acidosis effectively blocks some of the production of H^+ in eqn (A2.3), or it leaves some of the HCO_3^- produced in amino acid catabolism untitrated. Therefore, NH_4^+ excretion allows restoration of the plasma HCO_3^- and the excretion of the (dissociated) ammonium salt of a strong acid (the base might be Cl^-, SO_4^{2-}, or that of an organic acid such as aceto-acetate).

What happens in alkalosis?

(1) Ureogenesis is favoured
(2) Glutamine synthesis is depressed
(3) Glutaminase action in kidney is low
(4) Tubular luminal pH is high
(5) ammonium ion in urine is not detectable by the titration technique you are using
(6) the urine contains appreciable amounts of filtered HCO_3^-, which has not been reabsorbed.

What is happening in normal, control subjects? A normal diet is slightly acid. This is apparent for several reasons: first the pH of normal urine is low (usually 5–6), second, the titration reaction which unlocks the protons which have been buffered by HPO_4^{2-} usually reveals the excretion of some $25–50\,mmol \cdot day^{-1}$ of protons. There is also some ammonium ion in urine, perhaps $50–75\,mmol \cdot day^{-1}$. Some of this, at least, is probably being excreted as a response to the mild metabolic acidosis which eating an acid diet induces every day.

There remains a problem. Suppose the diet contains, on balance, a slight excess of dibasic amino acids, so that total catabolism of the protein yielded a 'not quite' equimolar amount of NH_4^+ and HCO_3^-? This ammonium ion would have to be excreted, as ammonium ion, to prevent it from causing an acidosis, as it would if it were used to synthesise urea. Does this mean it is not part of the 'total acidity' excreted?

There are other problems. What happens to acid–base balance if ureogenesis is driven at the 'wrong rate' relative to amino acid catabolism? What happens in renal failure, when the excretion of urea is impaired? It is by delving into the implications of this account of the origin of urinary NH_4^+, and of the stoichiometry of metabolism of ions released during the catabolism of foods, that we hope we might come to understand better the reasons for some of the consequences following from pathological disorders.

At present, it is traditional to work out the total acid excretion from a simple equation:

$$\text{Total acidity} = \text{titratable acidity} + NH_4^+ \text{ excreted} - HCO_3^- \text{ excreted}$$

If pH is less than 6.2, HCO_3^- concentration is negligible; above this value it becomes appreciable, and at pH 8, very substantial. Titratable acidity is the free and bound proton content of urine, and this is no problem conceptually. The excreted NH_4^+ remains a problem conceptually. It is not, strictly speaking, a way of buffering acid. On the other hand, it can be a very convenient way of producing what amounts to the (dissociated) salt of a strong acid combined with a weak base. It is also worth noting (see eqn (A2.2)) that NH_4^+ itself is an acid, albeit weak, and that although it is undissociated, it can reasonably be considered to be a route for excretion of acid, even though it cannot be regarded as a buffer for other acids.

For the purpose of this class, we are going to stick to the old formula, but remember that, one day, we might be proved wrong in assuming that all ammonium ion excretion is a consequence of a disturbance in acid–base balance. Part of ammonium ion excretion might be a pre-emptive move, to prevent such a disturbance from arising. If this proves to be the case, we may have to abandon the term 'total acidity' as it has been used for so long; the ammonium ion excretion would have no simple meaning, being composed of two elements, that which was excreted to prevent acidosis, and that which was excreted to promote recovery from acidosis. However, this debate does not detract from the meaningfulness of

changes in NH_4^+ excretion in your experiment, in which some subjects need to excrete alkali and stop excreting NH_4^+, and others need to recover from acidosis, and so excrete more NH_4^+. As it happens, in this class they are excreting the salt they first ingested, but by a very indirect route!

Ammonium ion: practical aspects. The ammonium ions that appear in the urine are formed in the kidney from the amino group of glutamine. These ions are, of course, present in the urine even before it is voided, but after urine has been passed it may become infected with micro-organisms containing the enzyme urease and additional ammonium ions may be formed in stale urine by the action of urease upon the urea present. For this reason, determination of ammonium ion concentration must be carried out on freshly voided or carefully preserved urine.

The ammonium ion may be estimated by a method similar to that used for the estimation of glycine. The method is based on the fact that when neutral formaldehyde acts on an ammonium salt, hexamethylenetetramine is formed and the acid previously combined with the ammonia is set free, e.g.

$$4NH_4Cl + 6HCHO = N_4(CH_2)_6 + 6H_2O + 4HCl \quad (A2.5)$$

The acid thus released can be titrated with standard alkali. Since, as mentioned above, glycine and other amino acids are estimated in just the same way, it will be appreciated that any amino acids present in the urine will be estimated as ammonium ion. In normal urine, however, the amino acid content is small and may be neglected.

Results
Your write-up should concentrate on the connection between theory and observation.

(1) Did per cent alveolar CO_2 move in the direction predicted by theory?
(2) Does excretion of an acid or alkaline load begin during the period of observations?
(3) Does urine pH reach its acid or alkaline limits?

(4) Does the rate of excretion observed account for a large fraction of the load ingested?

(5) Does the excretion of Na^+ change during the correction of a metabolic acidosis or alkalosis, and can you explain any changes observed?

(6) Do you observe an increase in urine flow of equal magnitude in all three experimental groups?

(7) What happened to NH_4^+ excretion, and why?

(8) Assuming that PCO_2 in urine at voiding is 40 mmHg (5.3 kPa), calculate the $[HCO_3^-]$ in your basal urine sample, and estimate the daily loss of HCO_3^- in urine, assuming a daily urine output of 1.5 litres at this pH and $[HCO_3^-]$. Is the daily HCO_3^- output of any quantitative significance?

Class data analysis: theoretical aspects

The data are analysed by computer which determines the **median** values. The advantage is that absurd results are almost ignored during the process of analysis, since gross errors gravitate to an extreme and have little effect in biassing the chosen estimate of the measure of central tendency. If means are used, this is certainly not the case.

The use of this technique markedly improved the estimated measure of central tendency from the first year in which it was employed.

By cumulating results over several years, the estimate can be steadily improved. The convergence of medians from the three subprotocols sampled in the basal condition (before inducing an acid–base disturbance) has been quite striking in each successive year. Furthermore, the trend of medians revealing what is happening during the class also becomes very clear.

For example, distinct changes in alveolar per cent CO_2 are seen in acidosis and alkalosis, despite the fact that the data has originated from students working largely without direct supervision using the Halane's tube. This technique is notoriously unsuccessful in general class use, and our students' individual data returns appear no better now than they were before this method of data analysis was introduced.

Urinary excretion of acids and alkalis: buffers

(Professor H. Britton, St. Mary's Hospital Medical School, London)

The purpose of this practical is to investigate:

(1) The excretion of acid and alkali by the kidney
(2) The properties of the bicarbonate buffering system including the effects of carbonic anhydrase
(3) The properties of the inorganic phosphate buffering system.

Most of our food is virtually neutral in pH yet in the process of digestion and metabolism acids and alkalis are generated which have to be excreted by the kidney. The purpose of the first part of the practical is to investigate how acid and alkali is excreted by the kidney and how this excretion is modified by diet. In preparation for the practical, students should read the Note — on the effects of foods on pH.

The bicarbonate buffer system is of major importance as a buffer in the body and is also involved in the urinary excretion of alkali.

The inorganic phosphate buffer system is unimportant in buffering within the body but its properties are of particular significance in urinary excretion.

Acid and alkali in the urine
The following measurements will be made on urine:

(1) pH
(2) NH_4^+ concentration
(3) Phosphate concentration and the proportions present as $H_2PO_4^-$ and HPO_4^{2-}.
(4) HCO_3^-
(5) Volume.

Procedure. All the students should provide a specimen of urine. The smallest appropriate beaker should be used, agitation should be avoided, and the reading of pH should be taken as quickly as possible to minimise the loss of CO_2.

Five volunteers are required, all of whom should have relatively acid urine (pH < 6): one will act as a control and should take

250 ml H_2O to ensure an adequate urine flow, two will take 100 mmol $NaHCO_3$ (8.4 g) in about 500 ml H_2O, and two will take 33.3 mmol (10 g) trisodium citrate (= 100 mmol Na^+) in about 500 ml H_2O. **The initial sample of urine from these subjects must be retained for further analysis.** The subjects should then collect their urine over 30 min periods for the following 1½ hours.

Analysis of urine. One student should be responsible for standardising the pH meter and supervising its use. Two students should be responsible for preparing duplicate blanks and standards for the ammonia determinations. The blank solution should be placed in a reference cuvette against which the unknowns will be read. Two students should be responsible for preparing blanks and standards for the phosphate determination. The blank solution should be placed in a reference cuvette against which the unknowns will be read.

Each subject should select a partner with whom he or she should be jointly responsible for the analysis of his or her urine as follows (see Table A2.1):

(a) *Measurement of pH.* Rinse the electrode and immerse in pH 7 buffer. If a pH of 7.0 is not indicated when the reading has become steady (use slight agitation), adjust meter to read 7.0 with the 'buffer adjust' control. Rinse the electrode, immerse in urine and read the steady value after *slight* agitation.
Make your readings without delay. Do not use strong agitation. (Why?) Do not knock the electrode which is made of very thin glass. If a series of measurements are made it is not necessary to standardise between each measurement.

(b) *Dilution of urine.* A 1 : 20 dilution of the specimen of urine should be prepared by adding 1 ml of urine using an Ultipipette to a 25 ml graduated cylinder. Fill to the 20 ml mark with distilled water. Cap with Parafilm and mix by inverting several times.
N.B. With some subjects a greater dilution may have to be used. If the optical densities in either the NH_4^+ or

phosphate (Pi) determination are much greater than standards consult the demonstrator.

(c) *Determination of ammonia* Place 100 μl (100 μl 'pipettor') of the 1:20 dilution of urine in a 15 ml plastic conical centrifuge tube. **First** add 2.5 ml sodium phenate reagent **and then** 2.5 ml sodium hypochlorite reagent from the automatic burettes provided. Without delay, cap the tube (plastic caps), mix by inversion, remove cap and incubate for 10 min at 55 °C. Blanks and standards should be prepared similarly with 100 μl H_2O and 100 μl of 1 mmol·l^{-1} NH_4^+ solutions respectively. Read the optical densities of the standards and unknowns against a blank with the Corning Colorimeter using a green filter (252/540).

(d) *Determination of phosphate.* Place 1 ml of 1:20 diluted urine using an Ultipipette in a 15 ml plastic conical centrifuge tube. Add 4 ml of ammonium molybdate in H_2SO_4 using the automatic dispenser and add 1 ml metol developing solution from the automatic burette. Cap with a plastic cap and mix by inversion. Allow to stand at room temperature for 10 min. Read against the blank between 10 and 40 min with the Corning Colorimeter using a red filter (252/600). Blanks and standards are prepared similarly using 1 ml H_2O and 1 ml of 1 mmol·l^{-1} phosphate standard respectively.

Plot a histogram of pH, NH_4^+, HCO_3^- and Pi against time. Divide the Pi blocks into HPO_4^{2-} and $H_2PO_4^-$.

(e) *Calculation of concentration of $H_2PO_4^-$.* From the appropriate Henderson–Hasselbalch equation for phosphate and the urinary pH calculate the ratio

$$[HPO_4^{2-}]/[H_2PO_4^-]$$

Let this ratio be r, then if (Pi)$_T$ is the total concentration of phosphate

$$[H_2PO_4^-] = \frac{1}{r+1}[Pi]_T$$

(f) *HCO_3^- content of urine.* Use the appropriate form of the Henderson–Hasselbalch equation for the bicarbonate system and assume a PCO_2 of 40 mmHg.

Table A2.1 *Grid sheet for entering experimental results (see text for details).*

RESULTS	Urine 1	Urine 2	Urine 3	Urine 4

Subject's Name . . . . took H₂O				
pH				
NH_4^+ mmol·l⁻¹				
Pi mmol·l⁻¹				
$HPO_4^{2-}/H_2PO_4^-$				
$H_2PO_4^-$ mmol·l⁻¹				
HCO_3^- mmol·l⁻¹				
Vol. ml·½hr⁻¹				

Subject's Name . . . . took NaHCO₃				
pH				
NH_4^+ mmol·l⁻¹				
Pi mmol·l⁻¹				
$HPO_4^{2-}/H_2PO_4^-$				
$H_2PO_4^-$ mmol·l⁻¹				
HCO_3^- mmol·l⁻¹				
Vol. ml·½hr⁻¹				

Subject's Name . . . . took NaHCO₃				
pH				
NH_4^+ mmol·l⁻¹				
Pi mmol·l⁻¹				
$HPO_4^{2-}/H_2PO_4^-$				
$H_2PO_4^-$ mmol·l⁻¹				
HCO_3^- mmol·l⁻¹				
Vol. ml·½hr⁻¹				

Table A2.1 *contd.*

RESULTS	Urine 1	Urine 2	Urine 3	Urine 4

Subject's Name . . . . took Trisodium Citrate				
pH				
NH_4^+ mmol·l^{-1}				
Pi mmol·l^{-1}				
$HPO_4^{2-}/H_2PO_4^-$				
$H_2PO_4^-$ mmol·l^{-1}				
HCO_3^- mmol·l^{-1}				
Vol. ml·½hr^{-1}				

Subject's Name . . . . took Trisodium Citrate				
pH				
NH_4^+ mmol·l^{-1}				
Pi mmol·l^{-1}				
$HPO_4^{2-}/H_2PO_4^-$				
$H_2PO_4^-$ mmol·l^{-1}				
HCO_3^- mmol·l^{-1}				
Vol. ml·½hr^{-1}				

N.B. This calculation should be regarded as approximate but will give a value of the correct order of magnitude. The errors arise because (1) the PCO_2 of urine may be appreciably higher than 40 mmHg and (2) loss of CO_2 from the urine before measurement of pH and alteration in temperature.

You should address the following points in your write-up:

(1) Comment briefly on your results.
(2) Do the effects of $NaHCO_3$ and Na citrate differ?

(3) Why might you wish to administer Na or K citrate to a patient?

(4) Why might you wish to administer $NaHCO_3$?

Titration of phosphate, action of carbonic anhydrase, titration of bicarbonate

The apparatus consists of a glass electrode connected to a chart recorder. Only two assemblies are available and the class should divide equally between them. For each titration:

One student should be responsible for the solution to be titrated.

A second student should be responsible for the additions. This student must make himself fully familiar with the operation of the 50 µl 'pipettor'. The additions must be made close to the surface of the solution so that all of the acid mixes with the solution.

A third student should be responsible for the recording.

Titration of phosphate. **Do not** adjust the controls on the amplifier of the pen recorder. Rinse the glass electrode with distilled water and immerse in pH 7 buffer. When a steady reading is obtained adjust the 'buffer adjust' control of the pH meter to read 7.00 on the digital readout. Verify that the pen of the recorder is accurately aligned on the midline of the chart.

Place 20 ml of 25 mmol·l^{-1} Na_2HPO_4 in a small beaker from the syringe provided. Rinse the glass electrode with distilled water and place it in the solution. When a steady reading has been obtained start the recorder at 3 cm·min^{-1} and make successive additions of 50 µl of 1 M HCl until the pH is less than 4. Mix after each addition with gentle agitation and note the steady reading on the digital display after each addition. **Do not knock the electrode**. Stop the paper, rinse the electrode and return it to pH 7 buffer.

Action of carbonic anhydrase. When CO_2 dissolves in water the hydrogen ion concentration rises and the pH falls. To slow down the rate of pH change and to make the action of the enzyme more evident a buffer may be added so that more hydrogen ions have to be produced for a given pH change. In the present experiment the nitrogenous base Tris is used as a buffer. It has a pK of $\simeq 8$ and thus buffers most strongly at around a pH of this value.

Place 10 ml of solution containing NaCl 120 mmol$\cdot$l^{-1} and Tris-HCl 20 mmol$\cdot$l^{-1} (pH 8.2) in a small beaker using the syringe provided. Ensure that the solution of carbonic anhydrase and a 20 μl pipette are available. Check that the display of the pH meter reads 7.00 with the glass electrode in the pH 7 buffer (if necessary reset the 'buffer adjust' control), rinse the electrode and place it in the solution of Tris buffer. Start the paper at 3 cm$\cdot$min^{-1}. When a steady pH is obtained bubble 5 per cent CO_2 briskly through the solution using the catheter tubing provided. As soon as the fall in pH has become linear (about 2.5–3 min) add 20 μl carbonic anhydrase solution (40 mg$\cdot$ml^{-1}) maintaining the CO_2 bubbling unchanged.

When the pH has reached a plateau, stop the paper, rinse the glass electrode with distilled water and return it to the pH 7 buffer.

Titration of bicarbonate. To a small beaker add 10 ml of a solution containing Na$^+$ 150 mmol$\cdot$l^{-1}, Cl$^-$ 125 mmol$\cdot$l^{-1} and HCO$_3^-$ 25 mmol$\cdot$l^{-1} using the syringe provided. (This solution is similar to extracellular fluid in tonicity and HCO$_3^-$ concentration. The concentration of HCO$_3^-$ is also the same as the phosphate already titrated.) Check that the display of the pH meter reads 7.00 with the electrode in pH 7 buffer and adjust if necessary. Rinse the electrode and immerse in the bicarbonate solution. Add 20 μl carbonic anhydrase solution (40 mg$\cdot$ml^{-1}). (The addition of the enzyme is not absolutely essential but the time for equilibration is appreciably reduced.) Now bubble 5 per cent CO_2 briskly through the solution using the catheter provided. (PCO$_2$ of 5 per cent CO_2 $\simeq 37$ mmHg.)

Note the pH when it has become steady. Add 50 μl 1 M HCl to the solution using the pipette and observe the changes in pH (since the volume of bicarbonate solution is 10 ml whereas the phosphate solution was 20 ml, the amount of acid added is effectively twice that in the corresponding additions to the phosphate solution). When a steady pH has been regained note its value. Carefully raise the catheter so that it blows gas over the surface of the solution. (This slows down gaseous exchange between the liquid and gas phases.) Add 50 μl 1 M acid and mix with **gentle** agitation. When the pH becomes steady and its value has been noted return the catheter to the solution and observe the change in pH. Record the steady value, repeat the procedure if desired and then make a series of additions of 50 μl 1 N HCl with CO_2 bubbling continuously, noting the pH after each addition, until the pH falls to < 3.5. Finally, stop the paper, rinse the glass electrode and return it to pH 7 buffer.

Results

Phosphate titration. Plot pH as a function of the addition of HCl (a vertical scale of 2 units per pH unit and one large division on the horizontal axis for each 50 μl addition of 1 M HCl are appropriate).

Answer the following questions:

(1) What are the ionic species of phosphate involved in the buffering?
(2) (a) What is the extent of ionisation of HCl?
    (b) What would be the H^+ ion concentration and the pH of the 20 ml of solution when 50 μl of 1 M HCl are added assuming no buffering?
    (c) What happens to virtually all of the H^+ ions that are added to the phosphate buffer?
(3) Write the equation defining the dissociation constant K for the phosphate buffer (a) in non-logarithmic form and (b) in the Henderson–Hasselbalch form.
(4) What is the approximate pK for phosphate buffer?
(5) Explain why the buffering becomes less effective (the slope of the curve becomes steep) at extremes of the curve.
(6) What are the proportions of the two forms of phosphate at blood pH (7.4)?
(7) In which parts of the kidney is phosphate titrated with H^+ ions in a similar way as in your laboratory experiment?
(8) How acid must urine be if phosphate in urine is to be excreted:
    (a) 90 per cent as dihydrogen phosphate?
    (b) 99 per cent as dihydrogen phosphate?
    (c) Can these pHs be achieved in urine?

Actions of carbonic anhydrase. Answer the following questions:

(1) What are the steps believed to be involved in the formation of hydrogen ions from CO_2 and indicate which step is accelerated by the enzyme?
(2) What are the proportions of the different forms of the bicarbonate buffering system at pH 7.4 and 37 °C?

Bicarbonate titration. Plot pH as a function of acid addition alongside the titration curve for phosphate. Use the same vertical scale for pH but each addition of 50 μl 1 M HCl should be separated by two large divisions along the horizontal axis since the volume of bicarbonate solution (10 ml) was one half of the volume of phosphate solution (20 ml). Answer the following questions:

(1) Explain the qualitative terms why the pH changes when 5 per cent CO_2 is bubbled through the solution.
(2) (a) From the calculation that you have already made in connection with the phosphate buffer (2(b) above), comment on the proportion of H^+ ions added as HCl that reacted with HCO_3^-. Is there a quantitative relationship between H^+ ions added and HCO_3^- broken down?
    (b) What has happened at the point where the pH falls very rapidly with the addition of acid?
(3) (a) What happened to the pH when the bubbling of 5 per cent CO_2 was stopped? What does this indicate about the concentrations of CO_2 and HCO_3^- in the solution? (Refer to the equation shown in the section on carbonic anhydrase.)
    (b) Why did the buffering become so much less effective when the bubbling of 5 per cent CO_2 was stopped?
    (c) When 5 per cent CO_2 is bubbling through the solution, the pH drops sharply when HCl is added and then returns slowly to a value near to the original pH. From your answer to 3(b) explain what is happening during the slow rise in pH.
(4) Write out the Henderson–Hasselbalch equation for the bicarbonate system in two different forms. What is the pK at 37 °C?
(5) The slope of the curve of pH versus HCl is a measure of buffering power, a flatter slope indicating greater buffering

power. From the appropriate Henderson–Hasselbalch equations explain why the buffering power of the bicarbonate system is so much greater than that of the phosphate system at the same concentration. Explain also why the greatest buffering occurred at the beginning of the curve with bicarbonate whereas it was midway with phosphate.

(6) HCl may accumulate in the body (e.g. because of the failure of the kidney to excrete acid). Thus, the addition of HCl as in the present titration has an exact parallel in life. However, an acidosis may also be produced by accumulation of the organic acids -hydroxybutyric acid and acetoacetic acid, or lactic acid. These acids have pK values in the region of 3.1–4.7. How completely are these organic acids ionised at physiological pH? How comparable would it have been to titrate the bicarbonate with these acids?

(7) The bicarbonate buffering system is normally the most powerful buffering system protecting the body against H^+ ions. In what respiratory condition would the effectiveness of this buffer system be very seriously diminished?

(8) In which parts of the kidney is bicarbonate titrated with H^+ ions in a similar way as in your laboratory experiment?

(9) What will be the concentration of HCO_3^- in the lumen of the kidney tubules when the pH of the tubular fluid is (a) 7.1, (b) 6.1, (c) 5.1. (Assume a PCO_2 of 40 mmHg)

Note: Effects of foods on pH

Most food is virtually neutral in pH but because of the processes of digestion and metabolism, the excretion products in the urine may be acid or alkaline. Usually the kidney has to excrete an acid urine.

It is of practical importance that urine is usually acid since if the ability of the kidney to excrete acid fails the hydrogen ions normally excreted will accumulate in the body and a metabolic acidosis will be produced.

Factors in food that make 'acid'

Phosphate diesters. Consider the phosphate groups in the nucleic acids

$$-R - O - P - O - R' - \quad + \quad x^+$$

with O above P and O^- below P.

Each phosphate group has one negative charge which will be balanced by a corresponding positive charge (X^+ = metallic cation or positively charged nitrogen). Hydrolysis to Pi will occur during digestion.

If the positive charge is K^+, after hydrolysis and absorption the following ions will be present in the body fluids:

$$K^+ + H_2PO_4^-$$

At pH 7.4, $H_2PO_4^-$ will ionise in the proportions shown

$$(1) \quad H_2PO_4^- \rightleftharpoons H^+ + HPO_4^{2-} \quad (4)$$

H^+ ions are therefore produced. These H^+ ions will be temporarily taken up by the buffer systems in the body.

$H_2PO_4^-$ is regenerated in the kidney by the tubular secretion of H^+ ions and is excreted with the appropriate cation (K^+ in this case). (How acid must the urine be to convert the majority of the phosphate to the dihydrogen phosphate?) Alternatively catabolism of the salts of organic acids taken in the diet may produce sufficient HCO_3^- to react with the H^+ ions as described in the following section.

Other phosphate diesters (e.g. ATP) behave similarly.

The nature of the cation X^+ is not important in the acid-producing process that occurs when diphosphate esters are hydrolysed. In fact, DNA in the cell is mostly as nucleoprotein in which the negatively charged phosphates are balanced by positively charged nitrogens in lysine and arginine. When lysine and arginine are catabolised these positively charged nitrogen atoms yield NH_4^+. Thus, the kidney excretes NH_4^+ as the cation and not K^+ as discussed above. For the carriage of NH_4^+ to the kidney see the section on ammonium chloride.

Sulphur containing amino acids. SH compounds are metabolised to H_2SO_4. Since sulphuric acid is a strong acid two hydrogen ions are produced for every SH group catabolised. These H^+ ions will be temporarily taken up by buffers in the body. The kidney cannot excrete H_2SO_4 as such. (Why not?) However, NH_3 is formed in the body from hydrolysis of peptide bonds (See Note below) and may be used to neutralise the sulphuric acid. Thus, $2NH_4^+ + SO_4^{2-}$ is excreted in the urine. Alternatively the catabolism of salts of organic acids taken in the diet may generate sufficient $M^+ + HCO_3^-$ (M^+ = metal ion) for the hydrogen ions to react with HCO_3^- and the salt $2M^+ + SO_4^{2-}$ to be excreted instead. (This may also happen if the subject takes HCO_3^- or citrates as in the present experiments.)

Ammonium Chloride. Ammonium chloride is **not** normally a major constituent of the diet. If a **large** amount of NH_4Cl is taken it is essential that the NH_4^+ be removed rapidly (Why?) and it is converted to urea (see Note below). Since urea is a **neutral** (uncharged) molecule this generates hydrogen ions. The overall reaction is

$$2NH_4^+ + 2Cl^- + CO_2 \rightarrow CO(NH_2)_2 \text{ (neutral)} + H_2O + 2H^+ + 2Cl^-.$$

Therefore, in effect, hydrochloric acid is formed.

HCl cannot be excreted as such in the urine. (Why not?) For excretion see the previous section.

Note. The majority of urea formed in the body is **not** formed in this way. The majority is derived in effect from NH_3 rather than NH_4^+ and hydrogen ions are not produced. 'NH_3' is generated in the catabolism of peptide bonds (—CO—NH—) and other **uncharged** amino or amido groups. Some of the 'NH_3' that is formed may not be converted to urea but may be used in the kidney to buffer hydrogen ions in the urine as described in the section on sulphur containing amino acids.

Smaller quantities of NH_4^+ will be converted to the transport forms alanine or glutamine. Considering glutamine, the reaction is

$$R\text{---}COO^- + M^+ + NH_4{}^+ + Cl^- \rightarrow RCONH_2 + M^+ + Cl^- + H_2O$$

glutamic acid   glutamine
(γ carboxyl shown)

where M^+ is the cation associated with γ carboxyl of glutamic acid.
The reaction of $NH_4{}^+$ with pyruvate to give alanine is similar:

$$NH_4{}^+ + Cl^- + CH_3CO\ COO^- + M^+ \rightarrow CH_3CH\ NH_3{}^+\ COO^- + M^+ + Cl^-$$

pyruvate   alanine

Thus, $NH_4{}^+$ taken up in either of these ways leads to the
formation of a salt $M^+ + Cl^-$ rather than HCl and hydrogen ions
are not formed.

In the kidney glutamine is probably the immediate source of
most of the ammonia in the urine. The amide nitrogen is first
removed by glutaminase but there is also further deamination and
metabolism of the glutamic acid that is formed.

Remember that urea is a neutral molecule

Factors in food that make 'alkali'

Sodium bicarbonate. Absorption of $Na^+ + HCO_3{}^-$ will increase
the $HCO_3{}^-$ concentration in plasma if $HCO_3{}^-$ cannot be excreted
rapidly enough by the kidney. By disturbing the equilibrium of the
bicarbonate buffer system, this renders the body fluids alkaline.

$NaHCO_3$ must be excreted in the urine. The $HCO_3{}^-$ concentration may reach $100\ mmol \cdot l^{-1}$ or more and the urinary pH may
rise to 8.

$KHCO_3$ and other bicarbonate salts will act similarly

Salts of organic acids e.g. K *or* Na *citrate.* Potassium citrate is
metabolised to $KHCO_3$ so its effect is the same as that of a
bicarbonate salt. Similar considerations apply to acetate, lactate,
β-hydroxybutyrate, aceto-acetate etc.

Note: Free organic acids (citric, acetic etc.) do not change in pH
because they are oxidised to CO_2 and H_2O, and CO_2 is lost in
respiration. Acid fruit juices consist of mixtures of the free acids

and salts and, paradoxically, fruit juices have an alkalinising effect.

Effect of a mixed diet
The pH of the urine and its NH_4^+ content depend upon the balance of the different factors in the diet. For example, metabolism of cysteine in the diet will give $2H^+ + SO_4^{2-}$ but fruit juices taken at the same time will give $K^+ + HCO_3^-$. Thus the urine will contain the salt $2K^+ + SO_4^{2-}$ rather than $2NH_4^+ + SO_4^{2-}$ or $K^+ + HCO_3^-$ which would have been formed if either had been taken alone. The urine may, therefore, be neutral in pH.

Questions
What is the effect of a meat diet on the urine?
What is the effect of a vegetarian diet on the urine?

Appendix 3

Problems

Department of Physiology and Pharmacology, Medical School, Nottingham

Objectives

The student will be able to:

(1) answer the questions:

How are acid–base disturbances likely to arise?

How effectively to the blood buffer systems function in man?

How do you measure the severity of an acid–base disturbance?

(2) assess the parts played by respiratory mechanisms and by the kidney in ameliorating the effects of several different disturbances.

(3) interpret laboratory measurements made on a patient who may have an acid–base disturbance.

Experimental disturbances

You should be able to work out the reasons why you might, with other deviations of the reported figures for arterial pH, PCO_2 and HCO_3^-, use the terms **respiratory** and **metabolic alkalosis**, and include or omit the qualifier **compensated**. You are invited to apply these terms appropriately in considering both the experimental and clinical disturbances below.

Try to work out the consequences of the following interventions in a human subject.

(a) The ingestion of ammonium chloride at a dose of $0.1\,g \cdot kg$ body weight^{-1} ($0.1\,g = 1.9\,mmol$)

(b) The ingestion of sodium bicarbonate at a dose of $0.2\,g \cdot kg$ body weight^{-1} $(0.2\,g = 2.4\,mmol)$

(c) Hyperventilating (a deep breath every 2 seconds) so as to keep alveolar PCO_2 below $2.7\,kPa$ ($20\,mmHg$) for 1 hour

(d) Breathing 7 per cent CO_2, 93 per cent O_2 for 60 minutes.

Your personal conclusions should be entered in a table (see Table A3.1) before consulting colleagues. Ask staff to interrogate your group when you feel you have got it right.

Use the Henderson–Hasselbalch relationship (as embodied in Figure A3.1) to analyse the four clinical cases in Table A3.2, writing brief answers to the questions for each column. Concentrate on giving short but discriminating statements. In particular, say whether the disturbance is in origin respiratory, metabolic or mixed, and whether it appears to be substantially compensated or not. Enter your personal conclusions before consulting colleagues,

Table A3.1 *Grid sheet for entering conclusions (see text for details).*

| Manoeuvre | Predicted Changes in blood | | Changes in urine |
	1° disturbance	2° response	
Ingestion of $0.1\,g \cdot kg^{-1}$ $NH_4{}^+Cl^-$. For $70\,kg =$ mmol of H^+			
Ingestion of $0.2\,g \cdot kg^{-1}$ $Na^+HCO_3{}^-$. For $70\,kg =$ mmol of $HCO_3{}^-$			
Overbreathing to hold PCO_2 $20\,mmHg$ for $30\,min$			
Breathing 7 per cent CO_2 for 1 hour.			

then make corrections if necessary. Ask a member of staff to interrogate your group when you feel you have got it right.

Table A3.3 gives three further clinical problems which may be used as an informal test by which you can discover whether you have achieved the objectives of the acid–base classes.

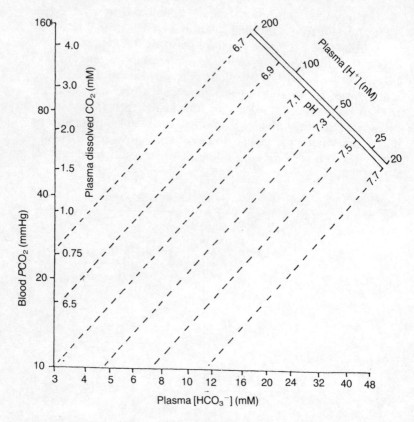

Fig. A3.1 Henderson–Hasselbalch relationship.

Table A3.2 *Grid sheet for entering conclusions for four case studies (see text for details).*

Patient, findings	Direction of disturbance	Type of disturbance	Likely cause
Female aged 26 on respirator in intensive care ward Blood pH 7.52 p_{CO_2} 29 mmHg Std. HCO_3^- 24 mM/L			
Female aged 75, known to be diabetic Blood pH 7.32 p_{CO2} 19 mmHg Std. HCO_3^- 9 mM/L			
Male aged 64, after resuscitation Blood pH 7.12 p_{CO_2} 54 mmHg Std. HCO_3^- 15 mM/L			
Male aged 17, semiconscious after sports accident Blood pH 7.32 p_{CO_2} 47 mmHg Std. HCO_3^- 23 mM/L			

Table A3.3 *Grid sheet for further clinical problems (see text for details).*

Patient, findings	Direction of disturbance	Type of disturbance	Likely cause

Index

acetazolamide 47
acetic acid, and CO_2 58
acid 97–8
  acetic, and CO_2 58
  amino, sulphur containing 143
  factors in food 141
  non-volatile 85
  organic, salts 144
  secretion of titratable 40
  solutions 2
  sources of in body 1–2
  strong 3
  urinary excretion of, buffers
    132–41
    urine analysis 133
  weak distribution 3, 51, 57–8
acid–base balance
  for the clinician 96–118
    diagram 100–2, 107–18
    history 96–7
    metabolic disturbances 100,
      105–6
    respiratory disturbances 100,
      102–4
  control in the whole body 75–93
    buffering in blood and
      extracellular fluid 78–81
    definitions in 76
    estimation of blood pH and
      pCO_2 90
    intracellular buffering 81–2
    management of disorders
      87–90
    physiological consequences
      76–8
    and cardiovascular system
      77
    importance of 1–3
    physical chemistry of 1–26
    and potassium 46–7
    problems in 146–50
    renal regulation of 26, 27–49
      compensation 44–6
    and sodium and diuretics 47–8
acidaemia 76–7
  respiratory 76
acidic disequilibrium pH 34
acidosis
  intracelluar changes in 67–8
  metabolic 30, 43, 48, 105
  renal tubular 45
  respiratory 45
adrenalectony 38, 48
alkalaemia 76, 77
  respiratory 76
alkali
  factors in food 144–5
  sources of in body 1–2
  urinary excretion of (buffers)
    132–41
    urine analysis 133
alkaline disequilibrium pH 35
alkaline solutions 3
alkalosis 128
  intracelluar pH changes in 67–8
  metabolic 105
  respiratory 45
alveolar ventilation 24, 25, 88

amiloride 48
amino acids, sulphur-containing
  143
aminophylline 108
ammonia, determination of 134
ammoniagenesis, renal 41–3
  inhibition of 43
  preduction and secretion 42
ammonium
  chloride 143–4
  ion, estimation of in urine
    125–31
anion gap, and bicarbonate and
  chloride 47
arterial blood, withdrawal of 90–1,
  103
asthma 107, 109, 110
Astrup (Copenhagen) 97

barnacle muscle 63–4
  photoreceptor adaptation 71, 72
base 3, 97–8
  deficit 76
  excess 76, 100
  weak 57–8
bicarbonate
  addition 85
  buffering system, manipulation
    of 18, 21–6
      transport of CO_2 in blood
        21–3
  chloride and 'anion gap' 47
  coupled and sodium
    reabsorption 37–8
  reabsorption of filtered 31–8
    basic cellular mechanisms
      31–5
        renal carbonic anhydrase
          33–4
        disequilibrium pH 34–5
    transport 35–7
    direct reabsorption 36–7
  sodium 144
  standard 100
  system
    excluding CO_2 loss from lungs
      14–17
    including CO_2 loss from lungs
      17–18
  titration of 137, 138–9, 140–1
  urinary acidification and
    restoration of depleted 39–44
Black, Joseph (Glasgow) 96
blood
  buffer systems in 13
  buffering in, and extracelluar
    fluid 78–81
  changes in 24, 25
  components, buffering power of
    20–1
  pH, estimation of 90
    electrode systems 91–3
    withdrawal of arterial 90–1
  transport of CO_2 in 21–3
body
  missing parts 180
  source of acid in 1–2
  source of alkali in 1–2
  scheme disturbance 180
  temperature, maintaining 122
  waste, eliminating 123, 124
  whole
    acid–base control in 75–93
    titration 82–7
Bohr effect 23
bronchitis 11, 112, 115
buffer 98–9
  mechanisms 2
  and pH 3–12
  solutions, effectiveness of 11
  systems in body 13–20
  in blood 13
  in extracelluar fluid 13
  in intracellular fluid 13
  in urine 13
buffering
  power
    measuring 12–13
    of blood components 20–1
    by proteins 18–20
  system
    bicarbonate 21–6
    manipulations of 18

carbonic anhydrase 22, 36, 37, 40
  action of 137–8, 140
  luminal 34
  renal 33–4
catheter 91
chloride
  ammonium 142–3
  bicarbonate and 'anion gap' 47
  shift 21
clinician, acid–base balance for
  96–118
CO_2
  and acetic acid 58
  addition of in titration 83–5
  and buffering power 62
  control of by respiration 24–6
  discovery of 96
  transport of in blood 21–3
crayfish neurones 66

data analysis 131
diabetic ketoacidosis 113, 116
diffusion trapping 41
disequilibrium pH 34–5
disorders, acid–base, management
  of 87–90
diuretics, sodium and acid–base
  balance 47–8, 106
doxapram 109

electrode systems 91–3
  construction 93
  glass 92
emphysema 111, 112
equilibrium potential for H^+ 55
  relative values of 56
extracellular fluid
  buffer systems in 13
  buffering in blood 78–81

food
  acid factors in 141
  alkali factors in 144–5
  effects of on mixed diet 145
  effects of on pH 141

glucose 1

glutamine 43
Great trans-Atlantic acid–base
  debate 101

haemoglobin 18–20
Haemophilus influenzae 111
Haldane effect 23
Hamburger shift 21
HCO_3^-
  increase in filtered load 29
  reabsorption of filtered 27, 32
Henderson–Hasselbalch equation
  3–8, 61, 101, 134
homogenate pH 50–1
hydrogen
  activity and concentration 98
  ion
    concentration, units for 3
    passive distribution of 53–5
    source of excreted 29–31
    urinary pH 30–1
  –sodium ion antiport 37–8
hypercapnia 44, 78
hyperkalaemia 46, 48
hyperventilation 104
hypocapnia 45
hypokalaemia 46
hypoxaemia 112

imidazole 19
imorganic phosphate 13–14
intracellular buffering 59–62,
  81–82
  and external CO_2 62
  importance of pK 59–60
  measuring power 60–2
intracellular fluid, buffer systems in
  13
intracellular pH 50–72
  buffering 59–62
  changes in ischaemia, acidosis
    and alkalosis 66–8
  external influences on pH_i 55–9
  H^+ ion as messenger 68–72
  methods for measuring 50–3
  passive distribution of H^+ ions
    53–5

regulation 62–6
ions
    ammonium, estimation of in
        urine 125–31
    hydrogen 3, 29–31
        concentration 3
        passive distribution of 53–5
        –sodium antiport 37–8
        as an intracellular messenger
            68–72
            activation of cells by
                fertilization 70–1
            barnacle photoreceptor
                adaptation 71
            membrane channels 71–2
        movements 57
ionic mechanisms 63
ionic (diffusion) trapping 41
ischaemia, intracellular changes in
    66–7
isohydric principle 99

ketoacidosis, diabetic 113, 116
kidney 27, 19
    rabbit tubule 67

Latta 97
leech neurones 66
luminal carbonic anhydrase 22, 36,
    37, 40

MacInnes and Dole 97
membrane potential 59
metabolic acidosis 30, 43, 48, 105
metabolic alkalosis 105
metabolic disturbances, in
    acid–base balance 105–6

nephron 28
neurone
    crayfish 66
    leech 66
    snail 58, 63–4
neutral solution 2
nikethamide 109
nomograms 70
    Siggaard-Andersen 80, 81

non-respiratory acidaemia and
    alkalaemia 76
non-respiratory pH 76
nuclear magnetic resonance
    (n.m.r.) ^{31}P 51–3

oedema, pulmonary 116, 117
organic acids, salts 144
O'Shaughnessy 97

Peters 97
pH
    and buffers 3–13
    Henderson–Hasselbalch
        equation 3–8
    values 8
    change 10–12
    disequilibrium 34–5
        acidic 34
        alkaline 35
    effects of food on 141
        acid factors in 141
        alkali factors in 144–5
        phosphate diesters 141–2
    intracellular 50–72
        equilibrium potential 55
        external influences on 55–9
        ions 55–7
        membrane potential 59
        snail neurone 58
        weak acids and bases 57–8
        H^+ ion as an intracellular
            messenger 68–72
        activation of quiescent cells by
            fertilization 70–1
        barnacle photoreceptor
            adaptation 71
        membrane channels 71–2
        intracellular buffering
            59–62
            and external CO_2 62
            importance of pK 59–60
            measuring power 60–2
    intracellular changes in
        ischaemia, acidosis and
        alkalosis 66–8
    intracellular regulation 62–6

ionic mechanisms 103
investigation of regulation 65
snail neurones, squid axon,
    barnacle muscle 63–4
vertebrate cells 64–6
methods for measuring 50–3
    homogenate 50–1
    indicators 51
    nuclear magnetic resonance
        51–3
    sensitive microelectrodes 53
    weak acid distribution 51
normal pH_i 53
passive distribution of hydrogen
    ions 53–5
measurement of in urine analysis
    133
non-respiratory 76, 85, 87, 101
regulation 123
    experimental procedure in 124
phosphate, inorganic 13–14
    determination of 134
    diesters 141–2
    titration of 137, 139
phosphofructinase 1
physical chemistry, of acid–base
    balance 1–26
pK, importance of 59–60
pneumonia 109, 111
potassium, and acid–base balance
    46–7
proteins, buffering by 18–20
protons 8, 9, 23
pulmonary oedema 116, 117

renal ammoniagenesis 41–3
    production and secretion 42
renal carbonic anhydrase 33–4
renal compensation of respiratory
    acid–base disturbances 44–6
renal control of acid–base balance
    27–48
renal tubular acidosis 43
respiration, control of CO_2 by 24–6
respiratory acid–base disturbances
    44–6
    renal compensation 44–6

respiratory acidaemia and
    alkalemia 76
respiratory acidosis 45
respiratory disturbances in
    acid–base balance 102–4

salbutamol 107, 109
Seldinger technique 91
Severinghaus and Bradley 97
Siggaard-Andersen nomogram 80,
    81, 102
snail neurone pH 58, 63–4
sodium
    bicarbonate 144
    concentration and output,
        measurement 125
    diuretics and acid–base balance
        47–8
    –hydrogen ion antiport 37–8
    reabsorption and coupled
        bicarbonate 37–8
solutions
    acid 2
    alkaline 3
    buffer 11
    neutral 2
Sorensen (Copenhagen) 97
spironolactone 48
squid axon 63–4
Streptococcus pneumoniae 109, 111
sulphur-containing amino acids 143

titration, whole body 82–7, 102
    addition of bicarbonate 85
    addition of CO_2 83–5
    addition of non-volatile acid 85
    lines 89
    non-respiratory pH 85–7

urea, as a neutral molecule 144–5
urinary excretion, of acids and
    alkalis (buffers) 132–41
    urine analysis 133
    urinary acidification and
        restoration of depleted
        bicarbonate 39–44
urinary pH 30–1

urine
    analysis of 133
    buffer systems in 13
    dilution of 133
    HCO_3^- content of 134–7
    titratable acidity and ammonium

    ions in 125–31
    experimental procedure
        125–30

Van Slyke 97
ventilation, alveolar 24, 25, 88